Deadly Innocence

Solving the Greatest Murder Mystery in the History of American Medicine

Nadine,

Thank you so much for your support, interest and truth, patients and love for family(?).

Best wishes for ongoing health, happiness and success.

Jen [signature]

1"/20/43

ADVANCE REVIEW COPY

1/2,500

II

ISBN: 0-923550-10-0

Additional copies of this book are available for bulk
purchases

for occupational health and safety training and employee
education programs, sales promotions, and premiums. Special editions, including customized covers, can be produced
in large quantities upon request. In addition, the post-expo-
sure follow-up forms reprinted in this book are available in
81/2 x 11 inch color coded, multiple copy format for em-
ployer-employee, medical-legal, and personal record keeping. For more information, please contact: Tetrahedron
Industries, Inc., 10 B Drumlin Road, Rockport, Massachusetts 01966, or call 1-800-336-9266.

Manufactured in the United States of America

First Edition

Dedication

This work is dedicated to my daughter Alena, and to keeping the natural loving innocence of children alive.

Leonard G. Horowitz, D.M.D.,M.A.,M.P.H., is an internationally known authority in behavioral science, patient education, and public health. Dr. Horowitz earned his D.M.D. from Tufts University, his M.A. in health education/healthy human development from Beacon College, and his M.P.H. in behavioral science/media health promotion from Harvard University.

Dr. Horowitz has held faculty appointments at Tufts University, Harvard University, and Leslie College's Institute for Human Development. He is the cofounder and *President* of Tetrahedron, Inc., a nonprofit educational corporation in Rockport, Massachusetts, and serves as a consultant to several corporations and public service organizations.

Dr. Horowitz has authored over sixty articles, seven books, and eight audiocassettes including: *AIDS, Fear and Infection Control, Overcoming Your Fear of the Dentist, Choosing Health For Yourself: A Clear and Practical Guide to Motivating Self-Care, Freedom From Desk Job Stress and Computer Strain*, and his most recent work *Deadly Exposures: If You Think You Might Have Been Exposed to AIDS or Hepatitis, This Book Will Save You Time, Money and Maybe Your Life!*

Dr. Horowitz is also an avid fitness buff and spends his free time hiking, swimming, snorkeling, singing, and playing guitar with his family. One of the most inspiring and captivating speakers in America today, Dr. Horowitz travels to more than one-hundred locations a year to present keynote speeches, lectures, seminars and in-service training workshops for groups of all sizes.

Contents

The Purpose of This Book

A cruel hoax has been played upon the American people. If you know anything about the story of Kimberly Bergalis, the first of six dental patients to receive the Acquired Immunodeficiency Disease Syndrome (AIDS) virus from Dr. David Acer, a Florida dentist, then you are just one more victim of deadly innocence. The United States Government's Centers for Disease Control (CDC), the U.S. public health care system, the media, and "mainstream" people just like you and I were all targeted by Dr. David Acer for our lack of awareness, sensitivity, support, acceptance, and caring about the victims of AIDS and the struggle to come to grips with the issues of being homosexual in a homophobic society.

If you find this hard to believe, you're not alone. In fact, after having put all the pieces of this extraordinary puzzle together, I find the entire "deadly innocence" affair totally unbelievable as well. The problem is it is frighteningly true, and the truth will be told herein. By doing so, this book is intended to be an immunization against the epidemic of infectious ignorance which has thus far plagued the American people regarding AIDS, the Florida dental tragedy, and the United States Government's role in perpetuating irrational fear for the sake of politics and profit.

The original purpose of this book was to shine a healing light of reason into the recesses of an irrationally frightened public's mind. My initial aim was to put the threat of getting AIDS from dentists, physicians, nurses or other health care workers into its proper perspective. I wanted to renew trust where it has been violated and dis-

charge the pervasive uncertainty people have about seeking routine health care, to enable clear and informed de-
cision-making regarding public policy development in
the age of AIDS. However, in the process of doing this
investigation, the book's depth and scope expanded. In
the end, I hope this work will alert readers to the extent
to which deceit is used and human life is sacrificed by
our nation's leaders to accomplish their political agendas.

Prologue

A smiling young dental assistant tucked a paper bib around Kimberly Bergalis's delicate neck. "Here this will protect you... the doctor will be right along. If there's anything we can do for you to make you feel more comfortable, please let us know." Kimberly smiled back.

A brief moment later, a lean, blond haired, blue-eyed, 36-year-old dentist entered the room. He walked to the rear of the dental chair where Kimberly sat. His right hand was anchored in the pocket of his white clinic jacket. His eyes fixed lifelessly on her for an instant then moved to the surgical tray at the back of the room. He took a step in that direction, then indifferently asked, "How are you feeling today?"

Before she could answer, his left hand reached toward the tools he would soon use to extract two non-impacted wisdom teeth from the pretty young woman's upper jaw. "I'm OK, Dr. Acer. How are you?" Kimberly responded.

After a moment of preoccupied silence he answered, "Fine." His left hand reached for the shiny silver syringe which lay among the gauze, suction tips, and other surgical instruments spread upon the tray.

While Kimberly gazed unconcerned out the window at the sunny lush Florida surroundings, Acer grabbed the syringe. He flicked his thumb against the shiny collar of the instrument and instantly drew back the plunger releasing the two inch glass tube of anesthetic. His right hand suddenly jerked from his coat pocket concealing a red colored replacement cartridge. The replacement was filled with his freshly drawn blood. He had drawn it the night before and refrigerated it to keep the virus alive. Deftly concealing the blood-filled cartridge against his right palm with his ring finger, he removed the anesthetic ampule with his free thumb and index finger and in a second he replaced it. The murder weapon was primed.

Holding the syringe in his right hand, he moved toward the innocent girl in the chair. Anticipating an assistant's intrusion he cleverly concealed the red side of the syringe by facing it down and away from the patient and the open door.

Acer's heart raced as he sat down on a stool behind and to the right of Bergalis. He reached behind Kimberly's neck to adjust the dental chair. With the touch of a button the executioner's chair began to slowly recline. The young woman gently fell back upon his lap.

"Now open wide."

His left hand moved behind the chair and reached around for Bergalis's jaw while his right hand moved towards her mouth holding the lethal weapon. He carefully rotated his wrist and "anesthetic" setup so the blood red side remained down and out of Kimberly's view.

The needle entered her mouth. Everything Acer had dreamed about and planned for eight weeks was happening. Without the slightest pause, as though rehearsed thousands and thousands of times, he pushed the needle through the soft pink flesh lining her inner cheek. Kimberly's body jerked and trembled slightly. Acer said nothing as he injected every visible drop of the deadly red liquid into her.

He then withdrew the syringe and quickly repeated the
ritual he had completed moments earlier, replacing the
spent cartridge with the one he had just removed. After
several more injections so that both upper teeth began to
numb, Acer turned his deadly gaze into Kimberly's anxious blue eyes. Then retreated from the room.

• • •

The above homicidal ritual was performed at least a
half-dozen times by Dr. David J. Acer between December,
1987 and July, 1989. These acts resulted in the deadliest,
most costly, and most publicized mystery in the history of
American health care. Despite years of investigative efforts
on the part of public health and criminal experts, the case
remained a mystery until now.

This is the complete story of the "deadly innocence"
affair—how and why David Acer intentionally infected
his patients, and why chief government investigators
from the Centers for Disease Control and Prevention
(CDC) and Florida Health and Rehabilitative Services
Department (HRS) failed to solve the mystery.

Herein lies an amazing story which confronts the
Clinton presidency and the two most powerful women in
American history with many critical and overlooked questions, which left unanswered, will continue to block
progress to true health care reform. This book should stir
public, political, health care, criminal justice, and social
welfare debate for years to come.

Introduction

By the time the American public became aware of the name Kimberly Bergalis, the tragic reality of what happened in Florida between Dr. David Acer, an unremarkable dentist, and his unsuspecting patients had become so distorted by government investigators and then the press that almost everyone was left feeling more anxious and confused about AIDS (particularly in health care) than ever. Health care workers themselves became prime suspects in the spreading AIDS epidemic. Patients' trust of dentists, physicians, nurses, and hospitals and blood banks fell to an all time low.[1,2] Health care professionals and public safety personnel, not immune to this "fear of AIDS epidemic," lost confidence, essential for career satisfaction, and much more.

The fear of AIDS became the American public's number one health care concern.[3] As a result, very conservatively, tens of thousands of people throughout the United States began suffering premature death and disease simply because they were too afraid to go for medical and dental treatments. Though it has been difficult to measure these public health and economic losses exactly, many experts recognized that following the CDC's report about the Florida dental tragedy, more people were probably dying from their fear of AIDS and their avoidance of health care than from the AIDS virus itself.

This tragedy continues years after the CDC began investigating the Acer case, because no one could explain exactly how and why it happened—until now.

In this book you will learn that Dr. David Acer planned for revenge to intentionally infect a selected sample of patients, six of whom have been identified at the time of this writing.

To amass the evidence, an investigator was needed who: 1) knew a lot about clinical dental practices, 2) knew enough about the epidemiology of AIDS to be able to critically evaluate the investigative data reported by the CDC, 3) understood human psychology and motivation, the keys to understanding criminal behavior, 4) was totally fed up with the toll the "fear of AIDS epidemic" has taken on the American way of life, our health care system, and our pocket books, 5) was practiced in the art of questioning authorities, and 6) had a little help from the Federal Bureau of Investigation (FBI). In essence, you either needed a well organized multidisciplinary team of health professionals and criminal investigators, which the CDC and HRS allegedly provided, or you needed a very unique individual. Dr. Len Horowitz just happens to be that person.

To set the wheels of truth and reason in motion, Len, a dentist himself, with masters degrees in health education/human development and behavioral science/public health, first needed to evaluate the authenticity of what the CDC and other authorities reported. During this review, he realized Acer's deadly transmissions could not have occurred the way the CDC speculated, and that perhaps the CDC had ulterior motives in reporting and omitting what they did.

To understand Acer's behavior and motives, this unofficial investigator needed to understand Acer's childhood, his personality, and the events which led up to his deadly deeds. This critical look into Acer's past will help

readers let go of their misperceptions about the man, and
the way in which the tragedy unfolded.

In summary, in order to solve this case—a tragedy
Lawrence Altman, AIDS reporter for the *New York Times,*
called "the greatest mystery in the history of American
medicine," Len had to establish: 1) that what the CDC
theorized happened in Dr. Acer's office to spread his HIV
infection to his patients could not have taken place; 2)
that the principal reason this case has remained a mystery was because the CDC failed to report the whole truth
about the case—in fact, you will learn that the CDC and
the HRS—conspired to keep vital facts about this case
hidden from the public; 3) the only way transmission of
HIV to six patients from one clinician could have taken
place was by intent; 4) there were powerful motives
which drove Acer to intentionally select and then inject
at least six of his patients with his HIV tainted blood; 5)
that Dr. Acer was capable mentally, emotionally, and
even imaginatively to devise and execute a murderous
plan to target the CDC, America's citadel of public health
and AIDS research, and humiliate them publicly and politically; 6) that the way in which Dr. Acer operated was
essentially identical to a very unique group of criminals
known to law enforcement authorities as sexual killers.

But Len didn't stop there. Driven by his desire to stop
the escalating death and disease brought on by people's
irrational fear of AIDS and health care, he continued aggressively researching scientific reports and news articles to try to understand what motives official
government investigators had in not reporting the whole
truth. This effort brought him to an incredible realization—that besides deciding it was in the publics best interest, the authorities held a firm belief in a frightening

public health and political agenda—one involving power, money and the future of American health care.

Though much of what is reported in this book is highly controversial and may offend and incriminate individuals in the highest positions of the United States government, it intended that a greater good will come from revealing the truth.

Thanks to Dr. Horowitz—for the sake of both scientific accuracy and public health—this book offers the truth about Dr. David J. Acer, the Florida dental tragedy, and United States Government conspiracy to cover it up.

Jackie (Lindenbach) Horowitz

The Key "Deadly Innocence" Affair Players

HIV Dx, Rx, and Tx
Paul Besong
Lab Technician
Frank Gutierrez, M.D.
Physician

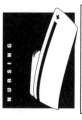

N U R S I N G

Mildred Gelfand, L.S.W.
Social Worker

AIDS Dx and Tx
Rolf Wolfrom, D.D.S
Oral Surgeon
H. Hoghooghi, M.D.
Pathologist

M E D I C I N E

Dr. David "Johnson" Acer

Family & Friends
Harriett Acer and
Victor Acer
Maureen Englebart
Edward Parsons

Independent Investigators
R. Runnells, D.D.S.
L. Horowitz, D.M.D.
J. Ostalkiewicz

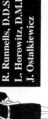

FBI
A. Burgess et al.
R. Ressler et al.

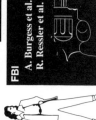

D E N T I S T R Y

Victims
Kimberly Bergalis
Richard Driskill
Barbara Webb
Lisa Shoemaker
John Yecs
Sherry Johnson
???

??? Political Players ???
HRS Secretaries Greg Coler
and Bob Williams
Governor Lawton Chiles
Janet Reno
Hillary Rodham Clinton

L A W

Deborah Sawyer, Esq.

Chief HRS Investigators
James Howell, M.D.
John Witte, M.D.
Thomas Liberti

GAO

Attorney General's Office
Robert A. Butterworth
Bruce Colton

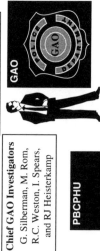

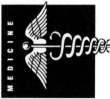

Chief CDC Investigators
Harold Jaffe, M.D.
Carol Ciesielski, M.D.
Nikki Economou, B.S.
Barbara Gooch, D.M.D.

RESEARCH
CDC
& HRS

Chief GAO Investigators
G. Silberman, M. Rom,
R.C. Weston, I. Spears,
and RJ Heisterkamp

PBCPHU

Chief PBCPHU Dental Investigator
Robert Dumbaugh, D.D.S.

TIMELINE OF EVENTS IN THE DR. DAVID ACER SEXUAL HOMICIDE CASE

Legend: Acer (open box) · Bergalis (gray) · CDC/HRS Personnel (hatched) · Official CDC Report (black) · News Media Report (black)

1985 — Acer

- **June:** HIV+ sex partner urges 36 year old Acer to be tested. He does not perceive risk, so he declines.
- **July:** Acer meets Ed Parsons, HIV+ male nurse who begins a non-intimate relationship with the dentist.

1986

- **July (Acer):** Acer begins to feel ill. Experiences chronic fatigue, intermittant fever, and diarrhea and notices swollen lymph nodes in right armpit.
- **August (Acer):** Seeks HIV testing/care @ Lauderdale; Uses alias/occupation. No sexual preferences est. with Dr. F. Gutierrez after HIV+ Diagnosis; reports 100-150 sex partners last 10 yrs.
- **December (Acer):** Dec. 3 exam w/ Gutierrez. Now ARC Diagnosis is established; "Safe sex" discussed during "State-of-the-art" HIV counseling. Acer continues risky sexual habits with other gays.

1987

- **February (Acer):** Feb. 13 exam with Gutierrez. Condition deteriorating; Still maintaining alias.
- **May (Acer):** May 6 exam with Gutierrez. T4 cell count =367 w 537-1571 normal; T4-T8 ratio 0.84 w/ 1.2-3.8 normal.
- **August (Acer):** Aug. 19 exam with Gutierrez. T4 cell count =286 w 537-1571 normal; T4-T8 ratio 0.6 w/ 1.2-3.8 normal; Diet and exercise prescription; Safe sex recommended.
- **September (Acer):** Notices KS on palate; Visits Dr. Rolf Wolfrom oral surgeon W. Palm Beach; Uses alias; Sept. 16, KS biopsy; Sept. 18, admits is homosexual Sept. 23 Case reported to PBC HRS AIDS dx on Sept. 30.
- **October (Acer):** By Oct. 5 Wolfrom learns Acer's true ID; Calls HRS again to report Acer is a dentist! (Also likely calls Dental Board).
- **October (CDC/HRS Personnel):** HRS complies; investigates; HRS DOH personnel interviews and exposes Acer.
- **November (Acer):** No further action taken by HRS 34 mos. later Acer's attorney says he got green light to practice from "authorities"; radiation tx for KS in Miami VA.
- **November (Bergalis):** Bergalis' initial exam by Acer on 17th.
- **December (Acer):** Dec. 17, Acer injects Kimberly Bergalis with his blood during "routine" "uncomplicated" wisdom tooth extraction visit.

TIMELINE OF EVENTS IN THE DR. DAVID ACER SEXUAL HOMICIDE CASE

	January	February	March	April	May	June	July	August	September	October	November	December
1988 — Acer	Jan. 17, Kimberly gets sore throat, enlarged tonsils w/ ulcerations, and enlarged cervical lymph nodes.		Acer receiving AZT treatment for KS which had spread to tongue, and a host of other symptoms; Acer feels a bit better.		Acer's oral cancer spreading. He seeks medical care at the VA Hospital in Miami.	June 6 to 20 Acer receives 2750 rads of radiation to treat oral KS. treatment results in mucositis.	Acer's KS responds well to therapy and tumors regress. Medical records show Acer fatigued but otherwise healthy.					
1989 — Acer	Acer plagued by respiratory illness and frequent coughing. He sees Gutierrez who notes he APPEARS SICK.	Acer begins to take step to sell dental practice. Lies to patients about having "cancer." Friend/ Employee M. Englebart knows truth, lies also to pts. and under oath.	Acer's now has recurrence of oral KS and it has spread to his abdomen and throax.		Acer uses electrical cautery unit to burn his oral KS lesions. (Had to be injecting himself at home with anesthetic to accomplish this without intense pain.) Acer calls mother to come to aid.	June 7, Acer hospitalized w/ pneumonia M. Gelfand records Acer's admission of "excessive drinking problem." He lies after stopping after AIDS dx. Accepts offer to sell practice;	Acer returns to VA hospital in Miami for lung treatments.	Acer sells dental practice to specialist	Acer sees Dr. Gutierrez who notices burned leasons in Acer's mouth; Acer finally admits to Gutierrez that he is a dentist.	Oct. 13, Acer sees physician Gutierrez for last time.		Dec. 14, Kimberly Bergalis hospitalized. Indian River Hospital reports "probably HIV infection" and AIDS to PBC-HRS	Kim is interviewed by Nikki Economou
1989 — Bergalis												
1990 — CDC/HRS Personnel			March 16, Kim interviewed by CDC-C. C. Ciesielski March 26, Kim interviewed by CDC and Florida HRS investigators and provides blood sample. Poor health now w/ pneumonia.	Dumbaugh of PBC-HRS investigates dental office. Acer refuses any more interviews. He hires attorney Deborah Sawyer to isolate himself from investigation		Acer flys to Ohio and Pennsylvania assisted by his parents to visit his siblings for the last time.	HRS investigator J. Howell interviews Acer re: letter to pts. Aug. 27, Acer goes to Jupiter Hosp. Enters PBC Hospice on Aug 31. Social worker records Acer couldn't express emotions.				
1990 — Official CDC Report							July 27, CDC's 1st investigation in MMWR. This fails to include vital info. e.g. dental staff interviews.		Acer dies on Sept 3rd Attorney Sawyer writes letter to patients published Sept. 6 & 7; Bergalis holds major News Conf. Sept. 22 Florida HRS reports B. Webb and R. Driscal's cases.	Oct. 1, CDC's report on investigation challenged by AMA, ADA, and other AIDS Research Groups. Organizations request additional information.	Nov. 11, Kimberly's story told on A Current Affair; Nov. 28, Defense's gynecologist examines Bergalis and files report she is not a virgin and has venereal warts.	
News Media Report												

Legend: ☐ Acer   ▨ Bergalis   ▨ CDC/HRS Personnel   ■ Official CDC Report   ■ News Media Report

TIMELINE OF EVENTS IN THE DR. DAVID ACER SEXUAL HOMICIDE CASE

1991

Acer

- **January:** Jan 7. Gov. Lawton Chiles appoints Janet Reno to head committee overseeing FLA. HRS; Jan. 18 CDC reports two more Acer victims: B. Webb and R. Driscall.
- **April:** April 5, 1991 CDC drafts Expert Panel Guidelines; U.S. GAO Begins Investigation of CDC's Investigation. April 5, 1991 blames HHS investigator who likely counseled Acer on continuing to practice, and "every one of you bastards [at the HRS] who knew Dr. Acer had full blown AIDS and stood by not doing a damn thing about it. You are all just as guilty as he was."; Cigna settles out of court with Kim.
- **May:** AMA Journal arrives in offices with research report showing most dentists do not believe CDC's investigation
- **June:** June. 14 CDC Releases MMWR report of L.Shoemaker and J. Yecs cases 4 & 5; June. 29 Florida Board of Dentistry mandates four hours of CE/AIDS prevention by Dec. 31.
- **July:** July 11, News: D.Lewis, U. of Georgia claims infections came from dental handpieces; July 30: NY Times reports CDC may ask for criminal investigation of Acer.
- **September:** Sept.26, Kim testifies in Congress. Am. Foundation for AIDS Research blames Bergalis hysteria on case and faulty CDC investigation.
- **December:** Dec. 8 1991, Kimberly Bergalis dies at her home in Florida.

1992

Bergalis / CDC/HRS Personnel

- **January:** Approximate time Ed Parsons presented testimony to Bergalis' attorney who then passed it on to HRS.
- **May:** May 15, CDC publishes definitive report on investigation in Ann int Med. Conclusions drawn are ludicrously inconsistent with available evidence. May 22 CBS and ABC T.V. shows cause handpiece hysteria.
- **June:** Harold Jaffee reports in NY Times Acer is deceptive/self-centered
- **July:** July 26, Montgomery, Bergalis, Webb, and Driscall attorney details case @ American Trial Lawyers Assoc. Becomes evident HRS and CDC might have been litigated w/ similar complaint.
- **September:** U.S. General Accounting Office reports that CDC's investigation methods were adequate. GAO's executive summary includes absurd explanation for the "mode" of [HIV] transmission from Acer.

1993

Official CDC Report / News Media Report

- **January:** CDC publishes definitive dental report on investigation in JADA. 9 co-authors now -6 are public health dentists. They edit May '92 article's absurd speculations and focus on safety of dental care.
- **April:** Dr. Robert Runnels, an infection control authority and expert witness in the Bergalis vs. Acer case publishes, AIDS In the Dental Office? Important information about Acer revealed.
- **May:** May 7, CDC publishes Update report on "Patients Treated by HIV-HCWs and relates to Acer case. No criminal investigation details provided or even suggested.
- **June:** Dr. Leonard Horowitz, a practicing dentist & behavioral science expert reviews Runnels' research and develops a personality profile on Dr. David Acer.
- **July:** Dr. Horowitz compares Dr. Acer's personality profile with those of 36 sexual murderers investigated by the FBI; there is an essentially identical match.
- **October:** Barbara Walters interviews Edward Parsons on 20/20. Provides additional testimony regarding Acer's malicious intent. Horowitz completes Deadly Innocence
- **November:** Horowitz holds press conference revealing evidence linking the Acer case with an HRS, CDC, and FL attorney general's office conspiracy- possible Clinton and Reno involvement

Legend:
- Acer
- Bergalis
- CDC/HRS Personnel
- Official CDC Report
- News Media Report

Chapter 1.
The Many Victims of Deadly Innocence

"Pinocchio, lies continue to grow until they become as clear as the nose on your face."

The Good Fairy,
Walt Disney's Pinocchio

I remember a time when I was about six years old. A neighbor's kid had thrown a rock through our picture window and my folks blamed me. No matter what I said, nor how I protested, I would be punished. My father rarely hit me, but on this unhappy occasion, he pulled his belt from his trousers and beat my behind until it was sore. At that moment, it occurred to me that adults can make wrong and harmful decisions. In response to this painful incident, I decided that it's wise to distrust authority figures—a decision which has gotten me into a lot of unusual situations. My investigation of the Dr. David Acer case is just one example. It's interesting that my distrust of authorities and urge to question things most people take for granted has made me one of them—an authority.

How does this relate to the case of Dr. David Acer? Like everyone, it would seem that Acer endured some painful childhood experiences. As a result he made some detrimental decisions about himself and others. These decisions affected the way he grew up and lived his life.

Though you might think the next few pages have nothing to do with the Acer investigation, you will see in the end this example illustrates the principles for understanding why Acer infected his patients and why we, in the United States, are currently witnessing an unprecedented escalation of social aggression and political corruption. Unless you understand this—that is, diagnose the problem—you are doomed to remain a victim of what I call "deadly innocence," as you will be unable to know the truth and choose differently.

By the way, I define "deadly innocence" to mean the innocence which makes you and everyone else, highly susceptible to being violated physically, mentally, emotionally, and spiritually. To the extent that our child-like innocence—violated or not—lives on in adults, you remain susceptible to those who would abuse you in body, mind, emotions and spirit. This is the source of all anxiety, neurosis, and even psychosis in the industrialized world.

The following are two simple examples which demonstrate the concept of deadly innocence and the etiology of psychopathology. The first is the most prevalent phobia in the United States, the fear of public speaking, and the second is the vast number of people who think of themselves as poor spellers. More than half of all Americans fall into at least one of these two groups. Let's see how these people's beliefs, attitudes and behaviors evolve and how childhood decisions can become self-fulfilling prophecies.

We'll use the story of little Mary Murphy. Mary is seven years old, in second grade. One morning the teacher announces, "Class, today we're going to do something new. We're going to have a spelling bee."

Mary, who's now sitting in the front row, gets very excited along with the rest of the class. "Oh, great," she and everyone else thinks, "A spelling bee, what fun!"

The teacher says, "When you come back from lunch this afternoon we'll begin." Everyone is delighted.

One o'clock rolls around and the teacher says, "OK class let's see how well you can spell." She turns to Mary and says, "Mary, please stand and spell Mississippi".

Mary stands and without hesitation begins, "M-I-S-S-S-S..."

Now what does the class do? Of course, everyone laughs. Would you consider this a painful experience for Mary? You bet it is. Mary loses her "self-esteem"—a valuable piece of her totally capable and worthy self gets ripped off at that moment.

Mary decides "I'll never stand up in front of this class again, I hate standing up in front of the class, and I must be a rotten speller." Now where does she go from here?

As the school bell rings, the teacher dismisses the class saying, "All right class, now listen-up, next Wednesday we're going to have another spelling bee, so study hard."

Next Wednesday rolls around, and with the fear of impending doom—another spelling bee—Mary begins to make new choices. First thing in the morning, Mary chooses to get sick, or at least she tells her mother, "Mommy, I can't go to school today, I don't feel good."

Her mom looks her over, feels her forehead, then says, "Mary, you look fine to me, why don't you run along and catch the bus."

So little Mary gets to school. How is she feeling? Right, a little nervous, nauseous and ill; she may even throw-up. In any case, she reports to the nurse. The nurse lets her rest on a cot for a few hours, takes her temperature and says, "Mary, honey, you look pretty good to me. Why don't you go to lunch, and then back to class."

Now it's one o'clock. How is Mary feeling? Right again, even more nervous. She walks into class believing that she's in trouble, consistent with her decision that she must be a "rotten speller" and doesn't want to be called upon to stand up in front of the class ever again. So where does Mary choose to sit? Right you are, in the very back of the room, which is like waving a red flag and proclaiming, "Teacher, here I am, I'm hiding from you back here so you won't see me or call on me."

Now, given the influence of reverse psychology, the teacher thinks, "Oh, look at that. There's little Mary hiding at the back of the room. I better call on her." Bingo. She calls on Mary.

Mary thinks, "Darn, I hate her."

Now how is Mary feeling? Right—as sick as a dog. She feels nauseous, very nervous, her palms are sweating, and her heart is beating wildly. Have you ever had this happen to you? Can you do anything very well when you're in this state? No—right again. So this time Mary is asked to spell the word "Arizona" and she spells it with a "q" instead of a "z" and again everyone bursts out laughing.

Many think and some say, "Boy, is she dumb... That Mary's so stupid... She can't spell worth a hill of beans... etc., etc."

Then there's that smart group of kids—the "clique" that Mary really wanted to impress. Now she overhears this peer group's leader saying, "You know, she's not only dumb, she's fat and ugly too." How is Mary feeling now?

Mary now lives her life feeling socially inadequate and she does her best to avoid all the situations, and deny the pain and loss, associated with her beliefs about how incapable, stupid, fat and ugly she is. To the extent that Mary thinks of herself as a poor speller, incapable of speaking in front of people, or even fat and ugly, these beliefs and negative attitudes take their toll on her social life, career, health and happiness. In essence, Mary may become emotionally scarred for life is she doesn't get help. To the extent she fails to reclaim the totally capable and worthy self she lost, she becomes a shadow of the person she once was or could have been. She is primed for a lifetime of anger, depression, and distrust of self and others.

By the end of this book you will see that David Acer had a lot in common with little Mary Murphy.

Mary's story demonstrates that childhood experiences involving pain and loss cause everyone to make decisions which may or may not be in our best interest or the interest of others. Mary now lives a large part of her life in fear, limitation and self doubt—not wanting to speak out, or to participate in class or with a certain group of people. She also grows to dislike any teacher that reminds her of the one who embarrassed her. She might even grow up distrusting all teachers and anyone else who represents an authority in her eyes.

David Acer lived most of his life in fear, limitation, and self doubt. Not wanting to speak out or relate to people socially, he became an isolated introvert. Acer did not believe he was capable of thinking and acting in ways that people would accept, so he simply withdrew—retreating into a fantasy world.

Mary's reference was what was said and done to her in second grade. Acer's reference was what was said and done to him during a troubled childhood. Both were innocent victims of social circumstances.

Your reference regarding AIDS and this mysterious case came from the media, including what you read in the newspapers, heard on the radio, or saw on television about Kimberly Bergalis and the other Acer victims. As a result of what you saw and heard, you likely decided that AIDS was a dreadful thing. You also likely decided that going for dental or medical care in the age of AIDS was pretty risky, particularly if your doctor happens to be HIV-positive. Your vulnerability in this decision making process was what David Acer preyed upon when he targeted you and the rest of mainstream American to become his victims—the victims of "deadly innocence."[1]

Chapter 2.
The Unofficial
Investigation Begins

Early July, 1990, a time when life seemed brighter for Democrats than Republicans. President Bush had just reneged on his promise to not raise taxes, and Democrats were celebrating.

"We've got a Republican Party that's coming unraveled," said Ron Brown, the national party chairman. The 1980's were "an extraordinarily unfortunate decade in American politics that has made the rich richer, the poor poorer and that has squeezed the very life out of the middle class."

Brown's aim—to make voters see the Republican greed, corruption and unfairness was behind the savings and loan fiasco and the short lived prosperity of the 1980's.

The sweet smell of victory in the '92 elections was in the air when the Democratic national committee met in Portland, Oregon to find Bill Clinton "stirring behind the scenes" as the principal presidential hopeful.

At the same time, on the other side of the continent, another story was unfolding—one which would have serious implications for future White House executives.

Late in the month, on July 27th to be exact, the CDC issued its first report to the world that a patient had become infected with HIV—the virus associated with

AIDS—by a Florida dentist. The information, published in the *Morbidity and Mortality Weekly Report*,[1] was picked up by virtually every news agency throughout the United States. Health professional organizations were at once placed on the defensive and challenged by media-driven fears about the safety of dental and even medical care, and the need for identifying health care workers with HIV.

At the same time, Dr. James Howell, chief medical investigator for the Florida HRS, was asking Acer through his attorney to help identify other infected patients. As a result of his requests Acer published an open letter to his patients on September 6 and 7, 1990 in newspapers throughout the state. The letter's content was a subtle but ghastly mix of information designed to not only "support" the CDC in their effort to identify more Acer victims, but also to disgrace the CDC through the national media, and send shock waves of fear throughout America.

Within three weeks of Acer's letter appearing in Florida newspapers, two additional patients who had been infected by him were identified—a grandmother, Barbara Webb, and a young heterosexual male, Richard Driskill. These cases were made public by the Florida HRS on September 22, 1990. As a result, the media fires burned hotter. Now there were three victims of Acer's deadly procedures.

The Webb and Driskill cases hit the news media even before the CDC had a chance to file their official report. Their update on these cases finally came four months later on January 18, 1991, in the *Morbidity and Mortality Weekly Report*.[2]

To make matters much, much worse for the CDC and organized health care in general, on September 7, 1990 Kimberly Bergalis, her lawyer Robert Montgomery, and her family held their first news conference. The event again brought national media attention that helped launch Kimberly's campaign to identify HIV-positive health care workers through mandatory testing and public disclosure. She ran this campaign nationwide from the Fall of 1990 through the Winter of 1991. Her crusade ultimately ended the following September, when she was seen as she appeared before congress—in a wheelchair, deathly ill—just two months before she died.

On the day most of the world learned about the Acer/Bergalis tragedy, I was in New York to meet with executives of a dental supply company. The purpose of this particular meeting was to determine the company's involvement in a national public education campaign initiated by the American Fund for Dental Health called "Oral Health 2000." Only minutes after the discussion began, it was decided that the most pressing issue in all of dentistry was the intense fallout that this case would have on the public's trust of dentists and dentistry. My expertise as a clinical dentist, behavioral scientist, and authority in patient education and fear reduction was immediately put to use. By the end of the meeting, I was assigned to develop patient and professional educational materials to help everyone feel better about dentistry in the age of AIDS. This was how I began my investigation of the Acer case.

Over the next year I worked feverishly to gain a better understanding of AIDS, its epidemiology, proper infection control techniques, and occupational health and safety standards that are required in dental and medical offices. I attended several AIDS education and training workshops including a very powerful and moving three-day program presented by the New England AIDS Education and Training Center, one of thirteen government sponsored groups dedicated to educating health professionals about AIDS patient care.

Within a year, I completed the patient and professional education materials I had been assigned to create, then traveled all over the United States presenting seminars to dental and medical teams to help bring rationality and peace of mind back to hysterical patients and insecure health care teams.

I conducted several patient and consumer surveys along with the help of my colleagues to find out exactly how people were responding to the uncertainty surrounding the CDC's reports about the Acer tragedy. After collecting this data and reviewing similar efforts by other researchers throughout the U.S., it became obvious to me that the CDC's inability to solve the mystery had created a deadlier epidemic than AIDS—massive and irrational fear and distrust of health care professionals. Although fewer than 40,000 Americans a year were dying from AIDS, our studies revealed approximately 2 percent of medical patients and 10 percent of dental patients who had been routinely receiving care, and as much as 24 percent of general consumers said they were avoiding even routine professional care due to fear of getting AIDS from their health care workers.[3] The hard fact about this revelation was that *at minimum tens of thousands Americans would suffer preventable death and disease in the coming few years due to their irrational fear of AIDS*—fear that had been largely instilled by the CDC.

My research revealed many inconsistencies between official CDC, ADA, AMA, and other health organization reports about AIDS, the Acer/Bergalis tragedy, and the alleged risks of transmitting HIV from one person to another via needlestick or other sharp instrument injuries.

For instance, Gabor Kelen, Chief of Emergency Medicine at Johns Hopkins University in Baltimore, Maryland, published a study showing the risk to health care workers of getting AIDS during patient care in his department where over 8 percent of patients carried HIV was one-in-a-million.[4] This was in sharp contrast to the study published by the American Dental Association telling dentists that their risk of dying from HIV patient care was a whopping 1 in 5,000—about the same risk of dying in a car crash on the way to work.[5]

As I searched the AIDS, fear and infection control research literature, I realized that more was unknown about this topic than was known and that the entire field was so vast that no one could truly be considered an expert though many were promoting themselves as such.

You might recall, for example, in July 1992, during the Eighth International Conference on AIDS held in Amsterdam, controversy raged about the possibility of a new strain of the AIDS virus which could not be detected. Newspaper and television reports throughout the United States were filled with warnings that a mysterious form of HIV was spreading. People became even more alarmed.

The mysterious illness is now known as idiopathic CD4 T-lymphocytopenia, or ILC. Lawrence Altman recently reported:

One hundred and eleven such cases, all but 10 in
adults, have been reported to the Centers for Disease Control and Prevention in Atlanta through the
first of February (1993).

. . . ILC is not new and not caused by any known
human retrovirus, and that it differs from H.I.V.-
infection epidemiologically, immunologically and
clinically.[6]

Most fascinating about the article, however, was an
analysis made by Dr. Anthony S. Fauci, Director of the
National Institute of Allergy and Infectious Diseases in
Bethesda, Maryland. His comments appeared in *The
New England Journal of Medicine* and suggested that the
syndrome probably has many causes. It was observed
that over 40 percent of those afflicted with ILC had risk
factors for HIV infection though no evidence was found
that the syndrome is spread by a virus or bacteria.[6]

What this report and most others failed to mention is
the great likelihood that HIV infection is not the sole
cause of AIDS either—the theory we were all led to believe.

Even the esteemed scientist who discovered HIV in
1983, French physician Luc Montagnier, now claims that
HIV infection does not necessarily cause AIDS. Likewise,
Dr. Peter Duesberg, a prominent American scientist, and
member of the National Academy of Sciences who first
mapped the genetic structure of retroviruses argues that
AIDS is not even an infectious disease!

How is this possible, I thought?

To be an infectious disease, traditionally, scientists
had to prove a cause-effect relationship between the suspected germ and the symptoms it is alleged to cause

when the germ spreads to others. These standards, known as "Koch's postulates," are based on three tests.

First, the suspect germ must be found in everyone with the disease. According to Duesberg and others, not all people with AIDS test positive for HIV infection. These patients would now likely be diagnosed as having ILC.

Koch's second postulate holds that the germ should not be present in individuals without the illness. Yet, of the approximately 1 million Americans who allegedly carry HIV, three-quarters have not developed AIDS. Furthermore, in a recent *CBS News* report, scientists noted that 8 percent of those who carry HIV antibodies have remained symptomless for over ten years suggesting that they may be doing something special to prolong their health. The reporters suggested positive thinking and good nutrition may be part of that special something.[7]

Koch's final postulate states that researchers should be able to reproduce the illness in laboratory animals using isolated germ cultures. With AIDS however, this too has proven impossible.

In the August 5, 1992 issue of *In These Times*, health writer Benjamin Goldman and AIDS journalist Michael Chappelle reported that defenders of the HIV hypothesis simply rejected Koch's postulates as being outdated. They stated that Harold Jaffe, the senior AIDS/HIV investigator at the CDC and Robin Weiss a British AIDS researcher argued:

> What seems bizarre is that anyone should demand strict adherence to these unreconstructed postulates 100 years after their proposition.[8]

Reporters Goldman and Chappelle, however, noted the advice of Nobel Laureate Walter Gilbert of Harvard University:

" Someone scientifically trained would not make that statement. Koch's postulates are an attempt at rigorous proof. If you cannot fulfill Koch's postulates, you've got a problem. You can deal with that either with hard thinking or with soft thinking. If you can block the virus and thus block the disease, that would constitute hard evidence that you were right." But in the absence of a successful treatment, Gilbert characterizes the attempt to dismiss Koch's postulates and fall back on incomplete epidemiological statistics as "soft-minded."[8]

The Politics of AIDS

My research taught me that the "HIV=AIDS" paradigm became entrenched in the minds of the scientific community as well as the general public beginning in April 1984. The U.S. Secretary of Health and Human Services, Margaret Heckler, called a press conference to announce that Dr. Robert Gallo, an internationally recognized researcher at the National Cancer Institute (NCI) had discovered the probable cause of AIDS. Heckler haled Gallo's discovery as "another miracle (in) the long honor roll of American medicine and science."

But the announcement was apparently designed more to meet the political needs of President Ronald Reagan than the human service needs of a country and world plagued by AIDS. Heckler called the press conference at a key point in Reagan's re-election campaign, when the president was being lambasted for not doing enough to fight the disease. Heckler used the photo opportunity to assail administration critics, saying: "Those who have said we weren't doing enough have not understood how sound solid scientific medical research proceeds." She then predicted that as a result of Gallo's work, a vaccine would likely be discovered by 1986.

Gallo claimed that over 90 percent of AIDS patients maintain HIV or antibodies to the virus. He then presented a theory which attempted to explain his observations. He speculated that HIV enters T-lymphocytes—the directors of the immune response—then freely reproduces itself therein. In the process, it destroys these key defense system cells which promotes opportunistic illnesses including infections and cancers.

According to the Goldman and Chappelle report, Gallo's hypothesis, "was a variation on his previous theories about the causes of cancer. Prior to the AIDS phenomenon, Gallo was a prominent player in the 'war on cancer' which President Richard Nixon launched in 1971."[8] That "war" closely foreshadowed the current battle against AIDS. "Just as Heckler predicted in 1984 that an AIDS vaccine would be available by 1986, spokespersons for the 'war on cancer' predicted a cure for cancer by 1976."[8] This false belief was again based on Gallo's theory that retroviruses caused cancer by invading the DNA of host cells, causing the cells to multiply rapidly.

Recently Gallo was convicted of scientific misconduct the article said. He apparently falsified the scientific documents he used to prove he had discovered AIDS.

Dr. Joseph Sonnaband, a pioneering AIDS researcher and founder of the American Foundation for AIDS Research, recalled the period following Gallo's announcement well. It immediately became clear to him that what

Gallo claimed as his discovery was actually the virus that Montagnier had identified a year earlier.

> I remember feeling sick to my stomach. I wanted to protest but all my colleagues told me just to keep quiet, and none of the scientific reporters seemed to see what was going on. In retrospect, that HIV was the cause of AIDS was certainly far from conclusively proven. But at the time, given the pressure and intensity of public fear, the newness of it all, and the glory of the new discovery, the American scientific community settled for less. The announcement was made and an industry was born... Gallo was certainly committing open and blatant scientific fraud. But the point is to not focus on Gallo, it's us. All of us in the scientific community. We let him get away with it. None of this was hidden. It was all out in the open, but nobody would say a word against Gallo. It had a lot to do with patriotism. The idea that this great discovery was made by an American.[8]

In another report, Sonnaband also voiced his opposition to the "fear of AIDS epidemic." Believing as I do that the fear campaign being waged by the CDC is more destructive than helpful, and that much of these anxiety provoking messages are directed at fund-raising, Sonnaband challenged everyone involved in AIDS research to focus more on patients. He stated, "So what have these hundreds of millions of dollars of research given us. Nothing! AIDS education? All I see is terror and confusion."[9]

I discovered numerous other reports generated by esteemed scientists who urged governmental officials to change the way they were waging their war on AIDS. The most logical to me was discussed in an editorial appearing in the November 1992 issue of the *American Journal*

of Public Health by Dr. Anke Ehrhardt, the Director of the
HIV Center for Clinical and Behavioral Studies at Columbia University in New York. Anke concluded the need
"to lay a foundation for prevention through behavior
change" could be met by targeting specific messages for
specific populations at risk.[10] A year and a half later, this
same recommendation was made public in a *New York
Times* article by Gina Kolata entitled, "Targeting Urged
in Attack on AIDS."

Kolata's discussion focused on the great success
some large urban cities throughout the world have made
in stopping the spread of AIDS by focusing their educational efforts on those most at risk. With AIDS currently
entrenched in many American cities, she wrote:

> Some experts are reaching a startling and controver-
> sial conclusion. They say the epidemic in the
> United States can be all but stamped out, even with-
> out a vaccine or wonder drug, by prevention efforts
> that zero in on 25 to 30 hard-hit neighborhoods
> across the nation.
>
> "We could stamp AIDS out," said Dr. Don C. Des
> Jarials, a drug-abuse specialist and AIDS researcher
> at Beth Israel Medical Center in New York and a
> proponent of a new approach. "I think that's a real-
> istic goal."
>
> Until now, most experts have held that because
> everyone is at risk of acquiring AIDS, messages
> promoting less risky behavior should be broadcast
> scattershot. Some of those experts still vehemently
> support that notion, saying that because AIDS has
> spread throughout the nation, it is fruitless to focus
> on a few neighborhoods.[11]

But many experts disagree with the status quo approach of frightening the public to prevent the spread of AIDS.

Kolata's article cited extensive new research which showed that:

> It is possible to reverse the course of an AIDS epidemic or even to prevent one if efforts are intense and narrowly focused. Such efforts have succeeded even among supposedly recalcitrant populations like intravenous drug users.
>
> . . . Jeffrey Levi, director of public policy development at the AIDS Action Council in Washington, said... "We need to communicate within a community about changing the norms of behavior," . . ."That's the piece that's been woefully missing since the beginning of the epidemic."
>
> Such an approach requires what Dr. Allan M. Brandt, a professor of the history of medicine at Harvard Medical School, calls "a reconceptualization of the problem—a fundamental rethinking of the epidemic."
>
> "The thing that leaps out at you is the way that almost every historical epidemic was socially, culturally determined," Dr. Jonsen said. People were not felled indiscriminately. "If you begin to think of that in terms of AIDS, you realize that the public concept of a virus that floats free and gets picked up almost at random" misses the point.[11]

That's interesting, I thought. *We're spending close to $15 billion dollars a year in the United States for AIDS patient care and AIDS research, and we've been missing the point and opportunity for prevention all along.*

After reading this, I began to question even more what I had read in the CDC's initial investigative reports about the Acer tragedy. It became inconceivable to me that five patients could have gotten AIDS from one dentist who had been routinely wearing gloves and masks.

I thought, *Maybe they decided to use this case to support their fear campaign?*

Chapter 3.
The Official CDC
Investigation

Background on the CDC and Florida HRS

The CDC functions as America's principal U.S. Public Health Service reporting agency, and it often joins state and local health departments in investigating unusual disease outbreaks. Through my involvement in public health dentistry, I knew that public health departments often work with very tight budgets, and they, along with the CDC often try to cut costs by sharing resources including personnel. Such was the case in Florida when the CDC and the HRS began to investigate the Acer/Bergalis tragedy.

The Florida HRS, on the other hand, is the largest state health and welfare agency in the United States. It now employs approximately 44,000 people and maintains an annual budget exceeding $9 billion. The organization operates from a central office in Tallahassee which directs eleven district units distributed throughout the state. The Palm Beach County Public Health Unit (PBCPHU) is one.

Both the CDC and state public health departments serve to investigate disease outbreaks and collect, report, and communicate relevant information about health risks and ways to prevent illness.

In 1981, approximately four years into the AIDS epidemic, the CDC directed all state health departments to collect and report data on AIDS cases in order to track the spread of HIV. So it was when Acer's case was reported and so it is today. State investigators of sexually transmitted diseases (STDs) are assigned to visit AIDS patientswho are unaware of how they became exposed. They ask questions as to how they became infected, identify sex partners, assist in partner notification, and help provide general information and counseling to assure personal support and public health.

The Investigation:
Superlative Science or Destructive Blunder?

On May 15, 1992, in the prestigious *Annals of Internal Medicine,* the CDC published its official report, entitled "Transmission of Human Immunodeficiency Virus in a Dental Practice."[1] As soon as I heard about the publication, I drove into Boston--to Harvard's Countway Library--where I had done most of my post-doctoral behavioral science research, to read the report.

As soon as I opened the journal to page 798 something very odd drew my attention. The article had more authors than any research paper I had ever read—eighteen to be exact. *That's bizarre,* I thought, as I considered the fact that the scientific community had recently been encouraged to use greater discretion in citing co-authors who had not made significant contributions to deserve the credit.

I noted the list of names; I recognized Dr. Harold Jaffe, and from my years of attending research conferences, Drs. Lawrence Furman and Robert Dumbaugh. The names and work of the other fifteen authors: Carol Ciesielski, Donald Marianos, Chin-Yih Ou, John Witte, Ruth Berkelman, Barbara Gooch, Gerald Myers, Chi-

Ching Luo, Gerald Schochetman, James Howell, Alan
Lasch, Kenneth Bell, Nikki Economou, Bob Scott, and
James Curran were unknown to me. In all there were six
physicians, five public health dentists, four PhDs, and
three BSs representing the Division of HIV/AIDS at the
CDC, the Division of Oral Health, National Center for Pre-
ventive Services at the CDC, the Florida HRS District IX,
the HRS central office in Tallahassee, the Los Alamos
National Laboratories, and the United States Public
Health Service.

Quite an impressive group, I thought, *maybe that's
why they added all the names.*

I immediately scanned the abstract and made note of
the conclusion:

> Although the specific incident that resulted in HIV
> transmission to these patients remains uncertain,
> the epidemiologic evidence supports direct dentist-
> to-patient transmission rather than a patient-to-
> patient route.[1]

I then read the first couple of paragraphs which indicated their purpose was to:

> Review updated epidemiologic findings which led
> to the conclusion that five patients of a dentist with
> AIDS were infected with HIV during their dental
> care...[and to] discuss the possible mechanisms of
> disease transmission.[1]

In a nutshell, the investigation showed that five patients (now there are at least six and possibly more)
treated by Dr. David Acer had become infected with his
particular strain of the AIDS virus. The investigators
showed that by reconstructing the patients' dental
records and treatments, they were able to determine that

the infections were unlikely to have been transmitted from one patient to another through the use of unsterilized instruments including dental handpieces (drills). They also noted the dentist did not have sex with these patients.

They discussed Acer's infection control methods and found that his sixteen staff members practiced a moderate level of infection control similar to most other dentists practicing at that time. The doctor and four chairside assistants wore gloves and masks during all "invasive" procedures, and no one, including the five infected patients, dental staff, and the dentist ever noticed anything unusual happening during patient care like Acer getting stuck, or bleeding into patients' mouths. They didn't even recall ever noticing any cuts or sores on Acer's hands.

Furthermore, for an AIDS patient, Dr. Acer apparently remained pretty healthy until close to the time he sold his practice. His medical history did not show common ailments associated with AIDS including:

> . . . thrombocytopenia or any other bleeding disorder, hand dermatitis, injury or dementia. No indication of peripheral neuropathy was present, although no record of a detailed neurologic exam or testing for neurologic dysfunction was found in the medical records.[1]

So how did it happen, I wondered?

The CDC investigators theorized:

> All five patients received multiple injections of local anesthetic, and a sharp injury during anesthetic administration could have resulted in contamination of the syringe apparatus with the dentist's blood, after which additional anesthetic

may have been injected into the same patient. A sharps injury could also result in direct contact of the dentist's blood with the patient's inflamed or non-intact oral tissues during the invasive procedures.[1]

This is absolutely ludicrous, I thought. When a dentist sticks himself with a needle during patient care, even during a difficult invasive procedure,[2] the first thing he would likely do is say "Ouch!" or at least flinch.

Most commonly, when this happens, procedures are momentarily interrupted for the doctor to de-glove, wash the wound, and administer first aid. Patients and chairside assistants almost always observe this and know something unusual happened. But *not one of Acer's six infected patients noticed any of this.* I was dumbfounded.

But I realized something even more ridiculous about this notion. I mused, *Could you imagine any dentist in his right mind* (Acer, according to the report, did not suffer dementia like some AIDS patients) *doing what they're suggesting happened? They want me to believe that a doctor, knowing he is HIV positive and his blood highly infectious, would continue uninhibited to stick a patient with the same contaminated needle he just stuck himself with? I also can't imagine anyone in their right mind continuing a procedure after slicing through his glove and skin and bleeding through the glove, into an open wound in the patient's mouth; all the while acting as if nothing out of the ordinary had happened. Is it possible that none of this would be observed by treatment assistants? No way, not in a million years!*

The report concluded,

Although the dentist began to routinely wear gloves in 1987, gloves do not prevent most injuries caused by sharp instruments.

That's true, I conceded, *but wait a minute. Gloves have been shown to significantly reduce the risk of blood-to-blood exposures after needlestick injuries.*

I recalled several months earlier reading a research study which showed--as common sense might predict--that as a needle enters or leaves a puncture wound, the latex or rubber actually wipes the needle surface moderately clean. Also, as a clinical dentist who had been stuck numerous times, while working with patients, I knew that following a needlestick injury through a latex glove, the blood usually pooled under the glove; *it never dripped out*--particularly not into the patient's mouth!

Sure injuries with thicker instruments can cause massive tearing of a glove and a lot of bleeding, I considered, *but had this occurred, Acer would most certainly have said "Ouch!" stopped the procedure, and his assistants and/or patients would have witnessed the interruptions. This whole thing just doesn't make sense.*

I continued reading,

All five patients had invasive procedures done after the dentist was diagnosed with AIDS and had evidence of severe immunosuppression... In addition, interviews with the dentist's health care providers and his office staff indicated that after he was diagnosed with AIDS, he frequently experienced fatigue, a factor which may have increased the likelihood of injury... There were multiple opportunities for the dentist to have injured himself during invasive procedures done on these patients, especially during periods of fatigue and ill health.[1]

Again, *if this happened,* I thought, *then why didn't someone notice it.*

Also, the CDC included root canal treatments in their list of "invasive procedures." This struck me as odd. In fact, they speculated that root canal therapy was the way two out of the original five Acer victims became infected (see Table 1 patients "E" and "G").

Though bleeding of the pulp of a tooth may occur at the beginning of a root canal procedure, I considered, *this lasts only for a very short time.* After thinking about it, I realized that it was virtually impossible in the context of accidental injury to have blood-to-blood transmission from doctor-to-patient through the twenty millimeter long canal of a tooth root.

Clinical dentists would understand this, but no one else, I realized. Only dentists who are in practice know the difficulty of getting thin root canal files and other tiny instruments into a hole slightly bigger than a pen tip, in a tooth being root canaled. *Accidentally dripping blood into such a small opening would be close to impossible,* I realized. *It would be like Michael Jordan hitting the hoop from behind the basket at the opposite end of the court!* My head shook in disbelief. *Could this really have happened two times in five patients?*

Finally, CDC investigators gathered some impressive research statistics about the likelihood of needlestick injuries happening to dentists. They reported:

In a survey of self-reported sharps injuries in 89 dentists, 32% reported 2 or more per month, and 3% indicated more than 15 such injuries per month. Another survey of 1132 dentists found a median of one sharps injury per month. Further although undocumented, the possibility that the dentist had a peripheral neuropathy cannot be ruled out; peripheral nervous system dysfunction has been noted in 9% to 35% of patients with AIDS.[1]

Very impressive numbers, I acknowledged. I thought about them for several minutes. Then it hit me. *Holy smoke! These statistics have nothing to do with the reality! They have nothing to do with evaluating the odds that 5 dental patients over a 18 month period, from December, 1987 to June, 1989, would accidentally get AIDS from their dentist.*

To understand the truth, people would have to understand the research on needlestick injuries and the rate of seroconversions to HIV (that is, becoming HIV-positive following an accidental exposure to someone's infected blood).

The truth, I realized, is this: the odds that a needlestick injury to Acer, presuming he would next carry the needle over to the patient, and stick them with his bloody needle is estimated to be approximately 1 in 280.[3] What does this number mean? It means from 1987 to 1989, Acer would have needed to stick himself *SEVERAL THOUSAND TIMES* for him to have accidentally infected five patients. Strange that no one ever noticed him getting stuck even once!

As I thought more about it, I realized that the CDC's HIV transmission hypothesis though plausible to the general public, and medical and public safety personnel was an insult to the intelligence of keen dental professionals.

That's probably why it was published in a medical rather than dental journal, I quipped. But I didn't realize how valid my jest actually was until nine months later. In January 1993, a similar article, written by essentially the same CDC investigators was published in the *Journal of the American Dental Association*.[4] This one however, did not include these incredible theories. *That's what I call intelligent target marketing!*

The Supervirus Theory

The CDC also considered and rejected the possibility that Acer carried what some call a "supervirus"--a highly infectious (virulent) strain which might have been easily transmitted. Dr. Robert Runnells, a dental infection control authority and author of *AIDS in the Dental Office: The Story of Kimberly Bergalis and Dr. David Acer*, and others had speculated this also.[5]

Their conjectures were based on the knowledge that such virulent viruses have been found to cause hepatitis. But the hepatitis virus is usually over a hundred times more infectious than HIV to begin with, and to date there is absolutely no evidence that this type of HIV has ever or will ever exist. According to the CDC report:

> Strain-specific virulence factors for HIV transmission have not been identified; further, no evidence was found to suggest HIV transmission from these patients to their sex partners...

> as might be expected had Acer's virus been a "supervirus."[1]

The Dental Handpiece Theory

That left the CDC having to consider just one last option, besides murder--the "dental handpiece theory."

One week after the release of the CDC's official investigation report, my wife Jackie, and I, sat glued to our
television, as did over thirty million other Americans.
We watched in horror on May 21, 1992, when CBS's half-
hour, special edition of *Street Stories* and then oddly
enough on the same evening by a *competing network*,
ABC's *Prime Time Live*--reported dental handpieces were
potential transmitters of death and disease throughout
the United States. The host of *Street Stories*, Bob
McKeown, began the report by issuing a warning.[6]

> The dental handpiece that's used to drill and clean
> your teeth, such as the ones used on Acer's patients,
> has become the basis for a new theory that should
> be a concern to virtually everyone who goes to the
> dentist... There's a growing body of evidence that
> the handpiece can be contaminated with blood,
> with saliva, with various kinds of body tissue. And,
> that unless this is properly sterilized between pa-
> tients, it can transfer bacteria and viruses from the
> mouth of one person to the next...[6]

The CDC, had days earlier, stated in their report the
contrary.

> It is unlikely that a high speed dental handpiece
> was used on [two or more] patients on any of the
> shared-visit days, and, to date, no studies have
> confirmed the transmission of blood-borne viruses
> such as HIV or HBV through the dental handpiece.[1]

"Who do you think the American public is going to
believe--the CDC or prime time TV?" I asked my intelligent wife rhetorically.

Jackie had been a dental assistant in my dental prac-
tice for six years, and before that she worked for the
Saskatchewan Dental Plan in Canada. I met her in
Mexico at the same time that I had been searching for

some office help. I not only found a great dental assistant, but a lifelong love and companion.

"All hell is going to break loose in the dental office tomorrow," Jackie predicted. Her intense blue eyes expressed serious concern. "This is incredible. People are going to be hysterical."

That's exactly what happened. As a result of the news shows, the demand for expensive dental handpieces skyrocketed. It took handpiece manufacturers and distributors over six months to catch up with backorders. The shows were associated with millions of dollars being made, literally overnight, by inside players, as handpiece manufacturer stock prices soared.

"Just another example of corporate America's control over the media?"

"Probably," Jackie responded, "How else could you explain the freak coincidence of two competing networks covering the *same* story on prime time on the *same* night?"

"Especially when the story was made public over a year ago," I reminded her.

I was referring to the report that had appeared in David Acer's hometown daily, the *Stuart News,* about dental handpieces on July 11, 1991. The report discussed studies performed by Dr. David Lewis, a University of Georgia research associate. The paper's editor, Tom Weber, had received a press release from Lewis who had been trying for over fifteen years to make people aware of the theoretic risk posed by unsterilized dental handpieces. The fact that Stuart, Florida, had been the hotbed of national concern about Acer made Weber take notice. He assigned staff writer Michael Cheek to cover Lewis's story, which was immediately picked up by the national press.

Dr. Lewis, who was criticized by the President of the American Dental Association for making reckless claims and leaking the story to the press before it appeared in a scientific journal, had made several unsuccessful attempts to gain support from the ADA and the CDC for his research as far back as 1989.[7]

Within a year, however, despite challenges to his professional credibility, scientific articles by Lewis appeared in *Lancet* and the *Journal of Clinical Microbiology*—two well respected scientific publications.[8] The ADA's position, thus weakened, was compelled (behind some state associations) to establish new guidelines for the sterilization of dental handpieces.

All the state and local dental societies and dental boards quickly followed suit, developing stricter guidelines and state laws requiring that all dental handpieces be sterilized. Compliance with strict handpiece sterilization and infection control guidelines added an additional five to ten dollars to the cost of every dental visit--an annual cost to the American public of over $17 billion. Dental manufacturers and distributors were the only ones delighted!

"It's probably a good idea, to sterilize all dental instruments that go into people's mouths," Jackie contended.

"Sure."

"So long as people know their dentists are using disposables and sterilizing their handpieces, they'll be safe."

"But how many people are going to know their dentists do this? How many are going to really feel brave enough to ask?" I said.

"You're right."

"They'll all be sitting there, looking all over the place, trying to find AIDS viruses in every corner of the room."

Unfortunately, I knew there were still many dentists who hadn't updated their infection control practices to meet the first series of OSHA requirements because of the time and costs involved.

"How do you think dentists are going to respond to these allegations?" Jackie asked as she got up to make us some tea.

"They'll wish they had bought stock in a dental handpiece company," I responded half joking while I thought, *most are still not going to buy this HIV transmission nonsense.*

Over the next six months I presented my knowledge and opinions about the news shows and CDC investigation to several thousand dental professionals throughout the United States. Just as I had suspected, only a small number of dentists really believed the reports. Dr. Barbara Gerbert, an expert in studying health professional responses to the AIDS epidemic, and her colleagues at the University of California, San Francisco documented this response and wrote that dentists were also suspicious about the CDC reports on the Acer case, and thought future dentist-to-patient HIV transmission was highly unlikely.[9]

Chapter 4.
Why the CDC
Ruled Out Murder

I learned from discussions with acquaintances at the CDC and other educational institutions that approximately eight months before the CDC and HRS investigators focused their inquiry on David Acer, he had sold his practice to a dental specialist. Essentially everything was then changed or removed leaving no evidence behind.[1] The absence of evidence at Dr. Acer's dental office allegedly made it very difficult for CDC and HRS agents to conduct a public health investigation.

In addition, according to their official investigation report, Carol Ciesielski, Harold Jaffe, and the others threw out the possibility that these infections were intentional due to a lack of evidence. They wrote:

> Interviews with family, staff, health care providers, patients and others who knew the dentist have not provided *any* support for this hypothesis. The dentist initially cooperated with our investigation. Additionally, most of the procedures done by the dentist were routinely observed by staff, all patients were awake during the procedures, and no unusual behavior was noted or suspected by either patients or staff members.[2]

Cooperative! My eyes bulged from my head. I couldn't believe I was reading this. I had learned during my research that *Acer only allowed one brief interview during which he answered questions.* If he hadn't, he would certainly have implicated himself as a murder suspect.

Equally suspicious was the fact that the authors' discussion contradicted statements Jaffe had made to the press eleven months earlier. Jaffe reported in a telephone interview published by the medical newsletter *AIDS Alert* that Acer's story was one of deception and self interest and that key documents in the case were inexplicably missing.[3,4]

When I spoke with other public health dentists around the country, most said it was fortunate for the CDC that Acer provided his blood sample, for if he had refused, the DNA analysis could not have been done, and the entire investigation would have been considered pure speculation. Acer would not have been incriminated at all.

"I can't believe they're saying he was suitably cooperative," I said to Jackie. "Why would they say such a thing?"

"Perhaps it wasn't so fortunate after all," my very pregnant wife answered. Maybe it was a set-up," she added.

"What do you mean?"

"Maybe the investigators overlooked the possibility that if he didn't provide some token support for the investigative effort he would have been under more suspicion himself."

About ready to tell my wife her hormones were affecting her head, I stopped. I instantly realized my wife was an avid reader of Robert Ludlum and John Grisham novels, and me—I've never read a murder mystery in my life. Given my obvious ignorance on the subject, I held my tongue.

"Say that again."

"Well it would have been highly suspicious of Acer, had he murdered his patients, to not cooperate at all—that would have implicated him the most.

"Yeah—I see that."

"They may have also overlooked the possibility that by providing his sample of blood for analysis it would have led the CDC into the trap of having to explain that indeed the virus came from him *somehow*!"

"Now you've lost me."

"Really smart killers know how to manipulate investigators, and lead them to dead ends. Maybe Acer was someone like that. You said yourself you believed he did it intentionally. He was a dentist, so he had to have some smarts, right? Then why not consider that he wanted them to know the patients infections came from him—somehow?"

Not quite sure of her logic, and not wanting to admit my ignorance, I simply responded, "I'll keep it in the back of my mind."

After dinner, I walked into the living room and sat back in my la-zy-boy recliner to consider the paper again. Jackie followed with tea and shortbread cookies—my favorite dessert.

"The CDC investigators reported that most, *though not all* of the procedures Acer performed were routinely observed by his staff." *I'm glad they clarified that.*

Dental assistants almost always observe and help with surgical procedures and the preparation and filling of teeth, however it is also common practice for dentists to inject patients within minutes of them being seated in the dental chair while the chairside dental assistant(s) is(are) out of the room cleaning, disinfecting, and/or sterilizing instruments used on previous patients or gathering the trays, instruments, and materials required for seated patients awaiting treatment.

"They didn't report that dentists are taught in dental school to hide the syringe from their patients while delivering the anesthetic to their mouths." I took a sip of chamomile tea and then continued, "When his dental assistants were out of sight, Acer could have easily reached into his pocket and withdrew a carpule which he had previously filled with his blood, insert it into a syringe, and inject it into his victims who sat awaiting their usual shot of novocaine."

"The entire process would have taken less than a minute."

"Preparing the murder weapon for use, behind the patient's back, would have taken him less than ten seconds."

"Scary."

More Overlooked Evidence

Over the many months I conducted my "AIDS, Fear and Infection Control" and "Dentistry in the Age of

AIDS" seminars I learned as much from the seminar participants as I did from my reviews of the scientific literature. The doctors would keep me on my toes by both asking good questions, and sharing golden nuggets of information which they had recently learned.

One common point of contention was that Kimberly Bergalis developed AIDS very quickly—within two years rather than the usual five to ten year HIV incubation period.

"There's about a 1 in 100 chance that this might occur,"[2] I explained to the groups. Then I would pull out a copy of the CDC's first *Morbidity and Mortality Weekly Report* on the Acer/Bergalis case published on July 26, 1990, which read:

> Time between the dental procedure and the development of AIDS (24 months) was short; 1 percent of infected homosexual/bisexual men and 5 percent of infected transfusion recipients develop AIDS within 2 years of infection.[5]

"This alone should have told CDC investigators that it was likely that Kimberly had been infected with a fair amount of blood. Microbiologists explain that disease transmission is based on three variables: 1) the host's resistance—Kimberly was a healthy young woman; 2) the virulence (strength) of the virus—if you remember, the CDC's investigation report indicated no evidence was found to suggest that it was a highly virulent form of HIV which Acer passed on to his patients. If it had been a super infectious strain, the victims' sex partners would have likely gotten the infection too; and 3) the number of viruses which got into Kimberly's system—the only unknown variable, had to have been pretty high."

"Clearly," I would add, "this is inconsistent with the theory advanced by the CDC. A large number of viruses being transmitted could not have occurred during an accidental needlestick injury since there are only about 100 AIDS viruses per milliliter of blood. An entire cartridge of dental anesthetic only holds 1.8 milliliters, a needlestick injury would have only exposed her to one or two viruses at most—possibly not enough to even cause an infection."

The most plausible explanations the health professionals attending my seminars agreed on was that Kimberly must have been injected with more blood than an accidental needlestick could render, or that Acer bled into her mouth for a fair amount of time, which could not have happened unless he really ripped open his hand and then kept it in her mouth for awhile.

"Since that was not observed, it probably never happened," I submitted.

One good-looking, middle aged doctor from Chicago shared, "Virologists and AIDS experts will tell you, that the quick death of Kimberly Bergalis is most consistent with someone injected with tissue samples containing live HIV, or someone having been given a very large dose of active viruses."[6,7]

"I can believe that."

Another doctor from Cincinnati exploded, "Were the CDC investigators blind? They reported that since no one witnessed any intentional exposures or saw anything unusual taking place when these patients were being treated that it couldn't have been murder. What an absurd conclusion!"

I agreed, "The fact that *no unusual behavior was noted or suspected by either patients or staff members* would not undermine the murder theory, it would support it!"

"Think about it," I concluded. "If you were Acer, and you wanted to kill a half dozen or more patients, would you be foolish enough to reveal your intent or methods to others who would undoubtedly try to stop you from doing it and/or would call the police?"

But the most disgraceful discrepancy I stumbled upon in my review of the CDC's May 1992 investigation report was the assertion that, "Interviews with family, staff, health care providers, patients and others who knew the dentist have not provided *any* support for this hypothesis."[2] Four months later I would realize that this statement was completely false when the General Accounting Office's investigation of the CDC would state that one person did provide support for this hypothesis.

Why the CDC chose to ignore this fact, and publish a falsehood became the question I asked myself countless times in the months ahead.

Chapter 5.
The GAO Investigates the CDC and HRS Investigation

By December of 1990, following the storm of publicity generated by Acer's open letter to his patients, Bergalis's national news conference and media tour, and the discovery of Barbara Webb's and Richard Driskill's infections, the CDC found itself pressed between public and professional demands. On the one side, organized medicine and dentistry was calling for more information and a faster investigation; on the other side, the public was demanding concrete answers and stricter controls. People wanted additional assurances about the safety of health care. The CDC found itself allegedly incapable of providing them.

At this point, several influential politicians and scientists criticized the CDC for not handling the case in an expedient or scientific manner. To calm this storm of discontent, in early April, 1991, Representative Ted Weiss, Chairman of the Human Resources and Intergovernmental Relations Subcommittee, Committee of Government Operations of the House of Representatives ordered the General Accounting Office (GAO) to review and evaluate the "methods and evidence" the CDC used to determine: 1) whether Acer transmitted HIV to his patients, and 2) how did the HIV transmissions occur? This review included an evaluation of all the information the CDC used to publish its official investigation report and its conclusions.[1]

The GAO report was published at the end of September 1992, and by the second week in October I had my copy. That evening after working in the dental office, having dinner, and helping Jackie bathe and comfort Alena, our beautiful three month old daughter, I sat back to read the report. Jackie, Alena in arms, joined me in the den.

I read out loud what the GAO investigators had written:

> There is no certainty regarding the mode of transmission. The most likely of several explanations is that the patients were infected through exposure to the dentist's blood. The dentist performed invasive dental procedures on each patient, and these procedures provided multiple opportunities for the dentist to have injured himself and then come into contact with the patients' blood. There is no record that the dentist became injured while treating these patients, however, and neither these patients nor the dentist could recall any such injuries.[1]

"In other words, the most 'likely' way it happened is that the dentist injured himself, and no one was around to witness it. Not even the dentist! If that isn't laughable, then you haven't got a sense of humor."

Jackie just shook her head.

"Listen to this. This is what they have to say about the intentional transmission theory:"

> No good evidence suggests that the dentist deliberately infected his patients. Substantial evidence exists that he did not...With the exception of one interview with an acquaintance of the dentist, the various interviews with the dentist, his family, dental staff, health care workers, patients, and other acquaintances provided no evidence that transmis-

sion was intentional... The dentist agreed to be interviewed by CDC and to have a blood sample taken for genetic sequencing. He wrote an open letter to his patients encouraging them to be tested for HIV. In this letter, written shortly before his death, the dentist stated that 'I am a gentle man, and I would never intentionally expose anyone to this disease...'[1]

"It sounds just like the CDC's report... but wait a minute. I remember the CDC's report said no one gave negative testimony against Acer. Here it says there was one exception." I read on for more clues and discovered that the:

> Acquaintance of the dentist, claimed in a deposition that the dentist may have been inclined to infect his patients in order to bring attention to the disease. This deposition was forwarded to the Florida HRS, and HRS personnel then also interviewed this individual. HRS in turn delivered the information to the Florida attorney general's office. Both offices determined that no additional action was warranted...the attorney general in Florida...declined to become formally involved, noting the absence of supporting evidence.[1]

I read this paragraph two more times, and then went on the next part of the report which said:

> The CDC did not bring a dental expert to its first, and only substantive, interview with the dentist. More detailed information about the dentist's practice (including his infection control practices and self injuries) might have been collected if such an expert had been present....a dental epidemiologist might have provided additional information about the dental practice that could have been helpful in identifying how the infections occurred...Because

this was the only interview CDC investigators held with the dentist, this oversight was particularly unfortunate.[1]

"My sentiments exactly! And it didn't take me a year and thousands of taxpayer dollars to figure it out!" I exclaimed.

Jackie sat quietly nursing Alena.

"I especially like the recommendation to hire a dental epidemiologist, but it's obvious to me that the GAO didn't practice what they preached. If they had hired a dental epidemiologist well-versed in the risk associated with needlestick injuries as well as the clinical practice of dentistry, they would have realized that their most likely mode of transmission was simply absurd! All of these possibilities are logically impossible."

I continued on my soap box as Jackie carried Alena now sleeping to bed. I followed closely behind.

"Scientists are not supposed to accept simply absurd or impossible explanations for observed events. They're encouraged to ask more sophisticated questions in order to get more reasonable answers. To think of more sophisticated questions they might have thought to look for additional clues in their own observations."

"Like the observation that the CDC report didn't mention the one exception," Jackie interrupted.

"Exactly, more sophisticated questions here would have been: 'What was this exception?', 'Why was it exceptional?', and 'How exceptional or great an impact might it have had?' I'll bet if they had asked these questions, they'd have probably gotten some pretty important answers."

"Will you tell me one thing?" Jackie questioned.

"What's that?"

"Why, if the GAO cited the CDC's failure to send a dental epidemiologist in on the investigation, didn't they also say something about the absence of a criminal investigator?"

"Explain."

Jackie continued, "Well, if this person—who was the one exception--provided information that incriminated Acer as a murderer, then why didn't they also note the failure of the HRS to involve a criminal investigator in their interview with this person? They said that HRS personnel interviewed the witness, not anyone from the attorney general's office. Don't you find that odd?"

"Good point," I acknowledged, as I moved closer to the table lamp for more light. "They did say that the CDC, through the HRS, involved the Florida attorney general's office in the evaluation of this person, and that 'both offices determined that no additional action was warranted.'"

"I wonder who the attorney general in Florida was who 'declined to become formally involved,' because of the absence of supporting evidence?"

"I'll call around tomorrow to find out."

"You must be tired."

"Yeah, I'm burnt."

"Why don't we go to bed, you know she's going to get us up early."

"All right, I'm ready." I turned off the lights and we called it a night.

The next morning, I telephoned the Florida attorney general's office. From employees there I learned that the GAO's report was apparently referring to Mr. Robert A. Butterworth. Butterworth became the chief attorney general in the state of Florida in January 1987, approximately nine months before Acer was initially investigated as an AIDS case by the HRS.

Chapter 6.
More Clues
Suggesting Foul Play

Between the Fall of 1992 and Spring of 1993, Jackie, Alena and I spent most of our time touring the country together in our thirty-two foot Southwind motorhome conducting seminars. Though we maintained a full, fast schedule, I considered myself pretty fortunate for being able to spend so much time with my family. Every day, Alena now almost one, was adding new skills and precious moments to our lives.

On May 1st, our family unit had to be separated when Jackie and the baby had to fly home. Our director of marketing had become very ill and Jackie was our only option for her replacement. So on this early Friday morning, with tears in our eyes, I took them to O'Hare Airport to catch a plane. As Jackie walked away with Alena in the backpack, Alena turned to wave "bye bye." My heart broke.

One week later, the first of two I would spend alone on the road, I was in Akron, Ohio. I was on my way into a Holiday Inn banquet room to present another "Dentistry in the Age of AIDS" seminar when my eye caught the front page headline in a *USA Today* paper box: "Sixth Acer Patient Identified with HIV."

I immediately recalled the scene from *Pinocchio* that Jackie, Alena and I had watched the week before. "You know Pinocchio," said the Good Fairy, "lies continue to grow until they become as clear as the nose on your face."

I chuckled to myself, not out of disrespect for the new victim's tragic fate, but because of the difference in consciousness between Walt Disney Productions and the Centers for Disease Control. I knew the truth had not been told in the Acer case, and at that moment wondered which person—Walt Disney or Harold Jaffe—was more fit to lead our nation's AIDS research efforts.

About a week later, newspapers across America carried interviews with eighteen-year-old Sherry Johnson, who had visited Acer at age thirteen, and her parents Johnnie and Suzanne. One, written by Robert Davis for *USA Today* interviewed Harold Jaffe about Johnson's case:

> " Why it happened in this practice and not in so many others is still a mystery," says Harold Jaffe, director of the HIV/AIDS division of the Centers for Disease Control and Prevention.
>
> Acer died in 1990. Another of his patients, Kimberly Bergalis, died of AIDS in late 1991.
>
> Bergalis and others had more invasive treatment, like root canals and tooth extractions, while in Acer's chair.
>
> The dentist cleaned Johnson's teeth and filled her cavities between 1987 and 1989. Such minor procedures sometimes require injections, raising questions about Acer's sterilization practices.
>
> Others infected by Acer are:
>
> • Richard Driskill, 33, of Indiantown, Fla., is quite ill, says his lawyer, Ralph Wiles.

- Barbara Webb, 67, of Palm City, Fla., is an ex-teacher who speaks on AIDS awareness.

- Lisa Shoemaker, 36, lives in Bloomfield Township, Mich.

- John Yecs has sued Acer's estate.

Jaffe says how HIV was transmitted by Acer may never be known unless "somebody comes forward who saw what he did or somebody the dentist told about what he did."

However, when Acer infected his patients, he changed the way health-care workers protect themselves and their patients.

Simple steps like wearing gloves and eye shields and using more strict sterilization techniques to prevent the spread of infectious disease have become more common.

"There is no question that this case has heightened the awareness of not only the public but the health-care profession about the meticulous use of precautionary measures,". . .[1]

Following these reports about Johnson's case, serious focus began centering on the possibility that Acer intentionally infected his patients with his blood. Until then, the CDC had been able to justify its conclusions that the transmissions of Acer's strain of HIV was most likely accidental— occurring during several invasive dental procedures that were performed by a fatigued or shaky Acer. Sherry Johnson's case was different—she never underwent invasive treatments by Acer, simply small fillings.

A *Chicago Tribune* article noted: "After factoring in the details of the Johnson case, many experts say the only theory that seems to fit all the facts is that Acer deliberately infected some of his patients."[2]

Former U.S. Surgeon General C. Everett Koop was among the first public health notables to go on record by stating, "We are left with no other conclusion than that Acer did it on purpose."[3]

University of Miami medical anthropologist and associate professor Doug Feldman publicly announced, "I think he took a needle and syringe, drew his own blood into it and deliberately injected it directly into his patients' mouths with the anesthetic."[4]

Intuitively I knew that all of these speculations were completely accurate.

The third week of May, I arrived back home, overjoyed to be reunited with my loved ones. After hugs and kisses to help make up for the two weeks of family deprivation, I noticed how much Alena had changed. It was as though she had become a little girl in my brief absence.

"I never want to be separated from you guys again," I said to Jackie. "This is what life is about and nothing is worth missing it."

Later that afternoon, I received a telephone call from Pamela Burt, the assistant editor of *Dental Office*. I had written numerous articles over the years for Steven's Publishing Company, the owner of *RDH* and *Dental Office*. She asked me if I had heard the news about Sherry Johnson and if I would write an article updating dental professionals about the Acer case investigation. She was particularly interested in what I knew about the CDC's continuing effort to unravel the Acer mystery.

My immediate response was, "I can do it, but you're not going to want to publish the things I have to say about the investigation."

"Why not?" she said.

"What I have to say is quite controversial," I replied.

"Oh no! That's just fine. I'm sure our readers would be delighted to learn what you know about the case."

I was about to say yes when something inside made me say, "Give me a day or two to think about it."

The next day I called an attorney who had been recommended to me by a friend. His advice was sound.

"Don't do it," he warned. "What you have to say is controversial and would be better presented in a scientific journal and not some throw-away trade magazine." He encouraged me to do some more research, find out what I could, publish a scientific article about the case, and then work with the magazines.

Sound advice, I thought.

Following another brief seminar tour in the Midwest, I began my review.

First I called a colleague who I met in 1981 when I spent the year as a faculty member and researcher at Harvard. My research involved studying self-care behaviors in grade-school children, and led to the discovery of "The Self-Care Motivation Model" for healthy and happy human development.

My colleague, a professional notable who wished to remain anonymous, stated, "Acer had destroyed or dispersed nearly all of his patient records prior to being investigated by the CDC. This made it difficult for the CDC to reconstruct Acer's patient records in order to determine whether two or more of the infected patients had been in his office on the same day, perhaps exposing each other."

We also talked about the value of confirming through blood testing and gene sequence analysis that Dr. Acer's patients were infected with virtually the same virus that Acer carried, meaning the virus must have come directly from Acer, not via patient to patient transmission. "That was the best part of the CDC investigation," the doctor noted.

"What about the murder theory?" I asked.

"There was some talk about Acer reusing syringes on the same patients and occasionally on different patients. The official report was published in the medical newsletter *AIDS Alert* from which excerpts appeared in a *New York Times* article written by Anthony DePalma, on June 26, 1991. The report stated that Acer had a habit of placing used dental syringes on a counter rather than on a special tray, and may have reused them."[5]

"Do you think it was wise for the CDC to decide against a criminal investigation on the grounds that no criminal evidence had been found?"

"The only investigation the CDC was capable of making was a public health investigation, which is vastly different from a criminal inquiry. The CDC had been chastised by the Government Accounting Office's investigators because they found that the HRS and CDC directors had neglected to involve a dentist during the initial part of the investigation and during the only interview they had with Acer."

"Yes, I read that."

"The worst problem," he concluded, "is that we are generating public health policies like OSHA regulations and infection control requirements based on one single cluster of doctor-to-patient HIV transmission cases, and we don't even know how they happened!"

"Is there anyone else who you can recommend I speak with regarding my investigation?"

"Yes, you should call Barbara Gooch. She was one of several public health dentists involved in co-authoring the CDC's report and the lead author of the official report published in the *Journal of the American Dental Association*."[6]

"Do you have her number?"

"No, but you can get it from the CDC."

"Thanks alot. Take care."

"No problem... bye."

After several attempts to make it through the maze of automated telephone answering system instructions at the CDC, I finally connected with Dr. Gooch.

Following my introduction, including my credentials as having been involved in dental public health and patient education for over a decade, Dr. Gooch told me, "I would like to speak with you, except I'm sworn to secrecy."

"Oh, really?"

"Before I can give you any information, you need to get a security clearance."

"How might I get that?" I asked thinking—*This is going to be a dead end.*

She then gave me the name of the CDC's press officer—Kaye Golan.

I called Ms. Golan immediately only to receive the typical snub any reporter might get from someone protecting valuable turf.

"We've already published everything we know about the case," Ms. Golan said. "However, if you would like, I can fax you copies of our previous reports."

"Thanks very much, I appreciate your help."

The next day I received her fax. Hoping the transmission would reveal something new and interesting, I surveyed it carefully. Unfortunately, I had already read all the material before—just as I thought—a dead end.

Then the fax line rang again. This time a copy of an article from the Knight-Ridder Tribune News Agency appeared. It was a clipping sent from Pamela Burt's office with the headline "Sixth dental patient to get AIDS virus fuels murder theory." The article, published on June 7, 1993, in the *Chicago Tribune* and *Denver Post* went on to report a few more specifics about Sherry Johnson.[2]

Again, Jaffe reported that Johnson's case "had certainly raised more questions about the possibility of criminal intent." All the other Acer victims had procedures that required the use of sharper instruments, Jaffe noted, while Johnson had just fillings. Jaffe and the article went on to report that the only two remaining possibilities being considered by CDC investigators were: 1) that Acer used teeth cleaning instruments on himself, then inadequately cleaned them before using them on patients, and 2) that Acer directly transmitted HIV to his patients through bleeding injuries to hands which then dripped into open wounds in the patients' mouths.

Basically the same position they took before, I thought.

The article also quoted Tom Liberti, the AIDS program administrator for Florida State's HRS, the person the article mentioned was in charge of the Acer investigation. Liberti stated,

> The only evidence we have to support the theory of criminal intent is the lack of evidence supporting any of the other theories...You have to fathom up some kind of scenario where he either draws his own blood or pricks himself with a needle every time...I can't tell you how many times I've asked the question: Did you ever see a syringe with blood in it? The answer is always no.[2]

What stuck in my mind was what one dentist had shared during my "Dentistry in the Age of AIDS" seminar in St Louis, Missouri, on May 26, 1993. He stated that his wife had come home the day before with a copy of *Globe*—the national tabloid published out of Boca Raton, Florida. He said the paper had quoted Sherry Johnson as saying she saw blood in the syringe Acer had used on her. The doctor lamented to the group following my speculations about murder, "You mean to say that we as dental professionals can trust the tabloids more than we can trust our own scientific publications?"

Unfortunately, I felt compelled in this case to answer, "Yes."

After reading the Knight-Ridder Tribune News Agency article, I jotted down Liberti's name and decided I would give him a call to ask whether he had ever questioned Sherry Johnson about seeing a bloody syringe. Three attempts to catch him between meetings over three days failed. In the meantime, I was able to secure a copy of the *Globe* article.

Quite frankly, I found the people who worked for the *Globe* to be extremely friendly and far more cooperative than anyone else I had requested information from during my research. The *Globe* librarian immediately faxed me a copy of the May 25, 1993, article, "Kim Bergalis's Dentist Injects Another Teen Beauty With AIDS"(38) and even called back to see if she could be of further assistance.

I wish the people at the CDC were as helpful, I mused.

The *Globe* article intimated that Sherry Johnson did say Acer had given her a "shot full of his HIV blood" but it did not appear to be a direct quote. She was quoted as saying,

> He always gave me a needle before telling me what he was going to do...He just did it and then he'd start drilling—but I could feel the drill on my teeth. He didn't numb me. That first shot had no effect. He'd only shrug when I complained about the pain and say: "Oh. I guess we'll give you a couple more shots, then." Then came the numbness.[7]

The very next day I was able to reach Tom Liberti who told me he could spare a couple of minutes.

"Thanks. I appreciate your time so let me get right to the point. I read your comments about the Acer investigation in the newspaper and I also read the comments allegedly made by Sherry Johnson about seeing a bloody syringe. Did you ever ask Sherry Johnson whether or not she ever saw a bloody syringe?"

His attitude, initially open, became guarded. "I'm not at liberty to disclose anything anyone has said to me during this investigation," he insisted. "Who are you anyway?" he asked.

After explaining my purpose, he simply stated, "The investigation is ongoing and I am unable to reveal who said what to whom, as it is all classified information."

"Well, thanks a lot for your time."

We hung up.

I can't believe this crap, I grumbled. *We people in public health are supposed to be on the same team.*

Chapter 7.
The Runnells Investigation

The day following my fruitless conversation with Liberti, a copy of *Dental Products Report* landed in my mailbox. I opened the cover, and there on first page I saw a full color display ad for *AIDS in the Dental Office? The Story of Kimberly Bergalis and Dr. David Acer* by Dr. Robert R. Runnells. I was delighted that Bob Runnells, one of four nationally known dental infection control experts had published a book about the Bergalis/Acer case. Anxious to get a copy, I immediately picked up the phone to place my order.

My first introduction to Bob Runnells was over the telephone in the late summer of 1991. Working as a continuing education program consultant for a medical and dental supply company in New York, I called Dr. Runnells to ask if he would be available as a speaker for the program I was putting together. I immediately found Bob to be a warm, generous, and most cooperative person. He not only agreed to participate as a speaker, but freely provided his professional expertise in editing the patient education materials I was preparing for publication. At the same time, Bob had been busy putting the finishing touches on an instructional videotape for dental office use entitled, "The Good Health Program," which I gladly viewed and critiqued for him. With a shared goal of educating patients and reducing the fear of

AIDS in dental offices throughout the U.S., we began a good relationship.

A few months later, in February 1992, I met up with Bob at the Miami Midwinter Scientific Session. He was there presenting an infection control lecture and I was there to distribute the educational materials I had developed. I presented Bob with several slides, I had prepared on the results of patient surveys my colleagues and I had conducted, showing the effects of fear on patients' behaviors and the need for more public education. Then we sat together during lunch to discuss the Acer case.

"Bob, I can't believe it was an accident or poor infection control," I said. "It just doesn't make any sense to me that all five patients could have been accidentally exposed to Acer's strain of HIV due to poor infection control or accidental injuries."

"No, Len," Bob responded as our waiter poured our water, "I believe that's just how it happened. Acer's infection control was abysmal, and as an expert witness in the Bergalis case, I can tell you there were many things he should have been doing that he didn't."

This was the first time I learned that Bob had been directly involved as an expert witness in the legal suits against Acer's estate, Cigna Dental Insurance Company (who sent the majority of victims to Acer) and CNA (Dr. Acer's malpractice carrier.) The suits were brought by Kimberly Bergalis, Barbara Webb, and Richard Driskill. Bob made no mention that he was writing a book about Kimberly Bergalis and David Acer, so when I first saw the book announcement, it not only caught my eye, but surprised me.

I immediately put through a call to Bob to congratulate him on publishing the work and to ask him if he had changed his mind due to the identification of Sherry Johnson's case.

"No, not at all" he replied. "The theory that Acer intentionally injected his patients is pure speculation. There's nothing to show that he would have done that...So many people have accepted that notion that they are coming up with all sorts of theories on how it happened."

"Then how would you explain Sherry Johnson's case when she didn't have an invasive procedure? Don't you think the facts of the case are better explained by the theory of intent?"

"I do not disagree with what you've said, Len. You can't prove or disprove the injection theory. But with very little hard evidence, all we can do is reconstruct the case based on oral testimony, and dig into what others have said about Acer. Acer's good friend Parsons was essentially the only one who said anything bad about Acer, and he is likely not to be trusted. By the way, another likely possibility is that Acer was carrying a super infectious strain of HIV. In the early days of hepatitis B we were not aware of this possibility either."

Since I knew from reading the CDC reports that they had ruled out the likelihood of a super infectious virus, I asked Bob, "Then would you say you disagree with the CDC's conclusions about the case?"

"No, I agree with them by-and-large. Acer, you must remember, was very ill and very fatigued. In this state he was much more prone to accidents. On top of that, Acer was a pretty sloppy person. And even though he was wearing gloves, gloving in 1987 was not the same as it is today. The gloves where much more fragile back then," he added.

"Well, Bob, I just ordered your book, and I'm really looking forward to reading it. I'll be working on an article based on my research, including this interview; after I read your book I'll give you a call if I have any more questions, and I'll be sure to send you a copy of my article as soon as it's ready. Thanks a lot for your time," I said.

"My pleasure Len. Stay well."

AIDS in the Dental Office?

A day later, Bob Runnells's book arrived. As I leafed through the book for the first time, I became very excited. There was a ton of data which hadn't been made public, including a good deal of information about Acer, his dental practices and philosophies and many of his personal habits, attitudes, and beliefs as discussed by friends, family, dental staff, acquaintances, and business associates. I read the 323 page book in less than two days—a feat for someone who failed the Evelyn Wood Speed Reading Dynamics Course.

Anyone interested in gaining in-depth knowledge about Kimberly Bergalis's personality and the emotionally moving struggle she endured is encouraged to read *AIDS in the Dental Office?*

Bob did an invaluable service to the American public by publishing what he knew about Acer. A true scientist and scholar, Bob recognized that others might interpret his data differently, and disagree with his conclusions, therefore, he invited the scientific community to scrutinize the work, and to continue the investigation in the hope of uncovering the truth and thereby benefiting public health. He ended the book by writing,

> The controversy will continue. The story is not yet complete, but...the lessons already learned from the tragedies of Kimberly Bergalis, David Acer and the others should not be ignored as the search for additional truths goes on.[1]

I devoured *AIDS in the Dental Office?* searching for such "additional truths." After reading it in its entirety, I then went back through it again, and highlighted all the information Bob had written about Acer.

Next, I took a stack of three-by-five notecards and made notes on the descriptive evidence Bob published about Acer's personality and behaviors including what Acer's friends, family, employees, and the CDC/HRS investigators had said about him. I then compared the information that Runnells, the CDC, and the news media had provided, and organized the stack of cards in two ways: 1) chronologically—analyzing the sequence of events which led up to Acer's identification as an AIDS case, his patients' infections, his death, and the CDC/HRS investigation; and 2) descriptively— noting the positive and negative adjectives people used to describe Acer.

After organizing this information on the notecards, Jackie and I sat up late every night for two weeks evaluating the information and trying to put the pieces of the Acer puzzle together.

Acer's Involvement Alleged

According to Bob Runnells, the investigation began on December 14, 1989, following the report of Bergalis's

HIV infection to the PBCPHU of the HRS by Indian River Hospital. As a result, the PBCPHU sent investigator Nikki Economu, who also worked in a dual capacity for the CDC as the AIDS Surveillance Manager for the State of Florida, to interview Kimberly Bergalis at her bedside.[2]

Following her HIV-positive diagnosis, Kimberly and her parents figured that the only possible way she could have gotten the virus was during her treatment with Dr. Acer. As a result, the Bergalis family urged the CDC to investigate Acer as the most likely cause of her infection. The experts answered that it was highly unlikely the AIDS virus could be transmitted in a dental office. Their comments were allegedly based on the fact that in nine years of record keeping, an HIV-positive health care worker had never been known to infect a patient with HIV.[2]

The CDC insisted that their investigation of Kimberly's personal and sexual history would reveal the cause of her infection. At one point they even insisted she was lying, and that her family was involved in the cover-up. One investigator had the gall to insinuate that her father had sexually abused her.

It took CDC investigators over three months, from mid-December of 1989 until late March of 1990, and tremendous expense to decide that Kimberly was a virgin, never used drugs, never received transfused blood, was not lying, and really believed her infection came from the dental office. Kimberly pleaded with HRS and CDC investigators to focus their investigation on Acer, but by the time they turned the investigation towards Acer it was too late.

Up Against a Liar

In late March 1990, HRS and CDC investigators began to investigate the AIDS plagued dentist. Unfortunately, Acer had now been retired for eight months, and he had sold his practice. It was therefore not surprising that when HRS investigator Dr. Robert Dumbaugh (the only dentist in the HRS who happened to be stationed at the PBCPHU) examined the office, little evidence of the former practice remained.

According to CDC reports, Acer alleged that he was too ill to undergo questioning. The investigators assigned to conduct and/or report on this first and only interview of Acer, medical physicians, James Howell, Carol Ciesielski, and John Witte, gained very little information.[3]

The following are excerpts from their summary along with notes on the numerous inaccuracies Jackie and I noted as we evaluated the report in late June 1993 on the deck outside our house.

> 40 year-old white male in a general dentistry practice since 1980. Prior to that, he was in the military.

" Runnells noted the correct date was actually 1981," I said to Jackie.

> History of hepatitis B years ago.

> Patient is bisexual.

" That's another dubious statement," I commented recalling from Runnells's book that "Acer's principal preference according to his gay friends was for men and *boys*."

Went to a counseling and testing site some distance away from his residence in 1987 *(Ft. Lauderdale)* and was shocked to have been HIV positive.

"That sounds like misrepresentation number two," I said as I pulled out a "Timeline of Events in the Dr. David Acer Florida Dental Tragedy"— a chart I had prepared to help quickly reference the chronology of events in the case (See "Timetable") Here I noticed, "The actual date was August 3, 1986, and it should not have come as a total shock to Acer that he was HIV-positive given the fact he was urged by an HIV-positive sex partner to seek testing in June 1985."

"Acer could have been living in denial," Jackie responded.

"You might be right. Runnells noted that Acer continued to practice unsafe sex even though he knew he was seriously ill and a risk to his innocent sex partners."

"That's in sharp contrast to the gay community's norms," Jackie responded. "By 1990 the vast majority of homosexuals had adopted preventive behaviors—apparently not so for Acer."

"The fact that he neglected to have himself tested for HIV after being warned about the likelihood of his infection as early as 1985, plus his disregard for the lives of his many sex partners appears to support your theory about him living in denial."

We had no idea how important this discussion and observation would become.

"Here, let me go on,"

He was told that his immune system was intact at
that time, but developed KS in September 1987.
Now has KS in lungs for which he receives chemo-
therapy. Has also had an episode of presumptive
PCP *(pneumococcus pneumonia.)* His physician is
in Ft. Lauderdale and he received medical care at
the Miami Veterans Administration Hospital.

He feels that he was infected through sexual activity, not occupationally. When his office is called,
patients are told he has developed cancer, but he
has heard that several people know that he has
AIDS. His parents have moved from Pittsburgh to
live with him.

He estimates that he had between 3,000 and 4,000
patients *(this was a stretching of the truth.)* About
800-1,000 saw him every 6 months or so. He was
one of the dentists on the state/county dental plan
(Cigna Plan); that is why CDC#242284 *(Kimberly
Bergalis's anonymous designation number)* sought
dental care from him. He estimates he had about ten
persons in his practice who may have had HIV
infection, and he was always 'extra careful' about
infection control practices when he did procedures
on these patients. He has worn gloves for patients
he felt were 'high risk' for years, but with the ad-
vent of HIV (can't remember exactly what year—
thinks it was 1987)—he and hygienists always wore
masks and new gloves for each patient. He did have
an autoclave but did not autoclave instruments after
every patient. He did not recollect details of the
infection control procedures, but said that prior to
the mid-1980's they used alcohol to disinfect equipment, but after HIV switched to recommended
'stronger disinfectants.'

"Runnells said that Acer was lying here. According
to his dental staff's testimony, alcohol continued to be
used as a primary disinfectant. In fact, Runnells wrote

that his practices were seriously "lacking in infection-control,"[3] I noted.

He does not recall any incident where he sustained a severe cut during a procedure. He does recall occasionally being stuck recapping the narrow gauge needle used to administer anesthetic, but said that usually the assistant would be the one to be stuck as she recapped the needle.

"That's not accurate either," I said, as I searched through the deck for the reference card. "Look, it says here, that according to staff interviews conducted by the CDC, 'only one seronegative staff person recalled sustaining an injury while washing sharp instruments, but no other specific incidents were reported by the staff.'"[4]

He sold his practice in the summer of 1989, and his office files are not organized. He had only one filing box at home with a few of his patient's dental records. The remainder of his files are scattered in many places—some are still in his old office (he suspects that the new office has discarded some), patients who have gone to new dentists have picked theirs up, and those in the state/county dental plan are in another office. His books were also disorganized, and he did not appear to have a patient roster. He did not have his 1987 appointment book.

"It is highly unusual for a well-run dental practice to be disorganized in the area of record keeping," Jackie remembered as a gust of wind blew her hair about her face.

"Especially a large PPO[5] provider like Acer," I added.

"Runnells also contended that 'Acer was not organized in maintaining records.' But I don't buy it; it just doesn't make sense," Jackie argued, now pulling her hair back into an elastic. "Acer, according to a CDC report, wrote finely detailed case notes. It seems to me that Acer's records were pretty well organized. His patients' charts had been separated and stored in various locations depending on their level of activity and required follow-up. For instance, charts holding accounts receivable, inactive patient accounts, and active patient records were grouped (by Acer, and in his final days with the help of his mother) and stored in various locations depending on the need to access them. Some records he kept in computer files (a high tech data storage and retrieval system,) others (those who owed him money) were located in his business office, and still others (those who required personal follow-up attention) were kept in his private office. The rest, his inactive patient records, were in the office storage room or at home—just like ours. I wouldn't say that was disorganized. I would call that organized."

"I'd agree."

Jackie continued, "Though the CDC made it a point to establish that Acer's records were very scattered, which made it difficult for them to be found."

"He could have scattered or discarded selected records and destroyed his patient roster and his 1987 appointment book intentionally to confuse investigators."

"Possibly." I said then reflected, "I can't believe that Acer, an intelligent, successful dentist practicing for over fifteen years would not know that the laws of Florida and most states require the maintenance of dental records for years after treatment is provided."

"According to Runnells's book, Acer informed the HRS investigators that a dental management company had instructed him to dispose of patients' records when they failed to respond to several recall notices."[6]

"That's unheard of in the dental management and consulting industry," I contended as I moved from the floor to a more comfortable position on the bench. "Instruction like that would place any consultant at risk for liability."

Jackie nodded in agreement, "So these statements by Acer defending the disposal of patient records could easily be another lie. Just another way Acer intended to confuse or mislead CDC investigators."

"You know something?"

"What?"

"I'm glad I married you."

"Well I'm glad you finally appreciate me after all these years."

Acer Cooperative?

After a kiss of mutual affection we continued the Acer analysis.

"To escape CDC inquiries, all Acer did was hire the services of Stuart, Florida attorney Deborah Sawyer. The report says that,"

> He had retained an attorney to deal with future interactions with CDC or the local health department.

"Right. According to Runnells, Sawyer and Acer's mother shielded him during the last five months of his life from HRS and CDC investigators and members of the press.

I pointed out, "Acer claimed he was too ill to undergo questioning. I believe that's lie number six. Even Harold Jaffe concluded that Acer's story was one of deception and self-interest."[7]

"Apparently, Bob Runnells and other investigators fell for Acer's deceptive sincerity when he claimed that this withdrawal into the safety of his home and family was so that he could die with dignity," Jackie commended while getting up to move back to the floor.

I continued, "No one in his right mind could think of dying with dignity knowing he had been the source of other people's HIV infections. A more humane and dignified response would have been to cooperate in every way possible to help the CDC discover the source of the mysterious infections."

"Good point."

"Acer was described by his very few friends and acquaintances as being very 'kind,' 'gentle,' and 'humanitarian.'[8-12] If this were his true nature, it is hard to imagine he would not have cooperated more completely with CDC investigators. Human beings would soon be dying from his actions, and he remained aloof.

"That's not normal behavior, even for a dying man," Jackie added.

I proceeded to make my case, "Consider in contrast Kimberly Bergalis, who was willing to leave her death bed to make a nineteen hour journey to Washington, D.C., to testify before Congress. She needed to be carried and wheeled from her home, strapped to a bed in a train, carried and then wheeled to the Congressional hearing room floor, and then returned home to die. And she did it all, not to clear her name, but to contribute to society."

Jackie brought up, "Remember, Acer did manage to fly back to Ohio and Pennsylvania to visit his siblings."

"When was that?" I pulled out the timetable and pointed to June 1990.

"More than two months after he told investigators that he was too ill to speak with them, and over two months before he died."

"The difference between Acer and Bergalis with regard to assisting authorities and serving the public was clearly one of choice then," Jackie concluded, "Acer was simply unwilling."

I finished reading,

We reviewed the dental records of CDC#242284 *(Kimberly Bergalis's number)* with the dentist who took over the county health plan, who has never seen the patient. The teeth were not impacted and this was a simple extraction of two upper wisdom teeth, which is a rather simple procedure requiring local anesthesia and dental extractors, which resemble pliers. He *(the new Cigna dentist)* told us that there was no indication from the record that anything unusual had happened, and that in general, he had been impressed with the level of documentation in CDC# 158093's *(Acer's)* charts.

" That supports my contention that Acer was a good record keeper," Jackie gloated.

"What else?"

"That's it for the report except that following the interview, Acer consented to have his blood drawn for viral analysis. The CDC then sent his blood to Los Alamos National Laboratory for viral sequencing to determine the DNA content or fingerprint of the virus."

"And that provided hard evidence that Dr. Acer's virus type was the same as Kimberly's?"

"Right. That left little doubt that Acer's blood had entered her body. "It seems clear as to how, the question is why?"

Chapter 8.
Will the Real Dr. David Acer
Please Identify Himself?

Over the long July 4th weekend, Jackie and I enlisted two deputies to our ongoing investigation. Barbara and Artie—two close friends who annually shared Independence Day with us in Rockport. I met Barbara as an undergraduate student at Rutgers College in 1971, and Artie, an engineer, was Barbara's significant other.

Barbara majored in psychology and earned her master's degree in social work. She worked for about a month counseling welfare clients, one whom shortly after their first session, committed suicide. Barbara's supervisor blamed her, at which point Barb decided she no longer wanted to continue her career in counseling. As an alternative career, Barbara began working for personnel placement services and now works for a large dental association.

Under two beach umbrellas set up to keep Alena out of the sun, I read through the deck of notecards describing Acer's childhood and tragic history. Barb helped provide psychological analysis while Jackie and Artie built sand castles for Alena to destroy.

"Dr. David Johnson Acer was born in Cleveland, Ohio on November 11, 1949. He was the elder of two sons conceived by Harriett Kullby and R. Johnson. Two years later, Harriet gave birth to a second son, Bruce. Unfortunately, for Harriet and the two young boys, David's father became extremely ill with poliomyelitis and passed away. I'm sure she felt the pressure of being a single parent with two hungry young boys to feed, and did her best to pay the bills and hold the family together."

"Excuse me," I shook a ton of sand out of my hair and off the blanket which Alena had thrown there. Then I continued, "Sometime after her husband's death she began to develop a relationship with an industrial products salesman named Victor Acer. She soon married him, and thereafter David assumed his stepfather's surname. Not wanting to let go of his blood father's memory, however, throughout life David used Johnson as his middle name (and as an alias when he wanted to hide his true identity.)

"Oooh, an alias. There's something strange about that," Barbara remarked.

"Runnells said he used it to maintain confidentiality," I explained. "The book fails to provide extensive details about Acer's childhood, but he did make several important observations. Here, listen to this one for example:

> Although his mother liked to emphasize David's independence and denied that she played a continuing close role in his life, David was protective of and dependent on his mother throughout his life.[1]

"It seems to me there's something wrong there," Barbara declared.

"Wait a few minutes," I persevered, knowing Barbara was never short on words, and if I didn't get through his childhood, we'd never get to discuss his adult life. "We'll talk about it."

"Together Harriett and Victor had two more children, a girl named Cynthia and a new little brother Kenneth. The family lived in Kirtland, Ohio, a Cleveland suburb, for a time, and then moved to Canton, Ohio, where David attended Hoover High School. He was remembered as a quiet student whose activities included the yearbook staff, the German Club and the wrestling team."

"It's interesting that he'd choose to participate, as a young homosexual, in the most rugged, maximum male body contact sport—wrestling," Jackie added as she perfectly set a sand bear formation down in front of Alena.

"A choice quite befitting a gay young man whose parents disapproved of mama's boys," I responded then continued reading the next card.[1]

"David's health history included the usual childhood illnesses, a few strep throat infections, wisdom teeth extraction at the age of twenty, and hepatitis B infection."[1]

"It's very interesting that Acer would be diagnosed with hepatitis B infection at age twenty, right around the time he had his wisdom teeth removed," I said to the group. "Hepatitis B infection is principally a sexually transmitted disease, most commonly spread through unprotected sex among homosexual males or individuals with multiple sex partners. It can also be spread through the use of contaminated surgical instruments such as those which may have been used on David by an oral surgeon practicing in 1969 before the days of strict infection control. It is possible that Acer's dental surgeon infected him with hepatitis at age twenty which might have given Acer the idea of infecting his patients with HIV."

"Or more likely," added Barbara "he had already established promiscuous and risky sexual habits by the end of high school."

"That's conceivable," I said and continued reading.

"After graduating from high school, the six-foot, 175 pound Acer made plans to attend Ohio State University where he received his undergraduate pre-dental degree and then his dental doctorate, carrying a B average throughout. His professors and classmates remembered Acer as being sandy haired, thin, shy, quiet, unremarkable, studious, someone who wouldn't hurt anything, a loner and content unto himself."[1]

"After a two-year stint in the Air Force Dental Corps serving in Germany, he returned to fulfill his military commitment in Shreveport, Louisiana. At the end of the year, he was honorably discharged and moved to Florida."

"After establishing himself in Florida as a licensed dentist, Acer joined a growing dental service company in Opa-locka, which later became known as CIGNA Dental Health of Florida, Incorporated. The company was headed by a very successful dentist, Dr. Larry Brody, who taught Acer a lot about the business of running a large dental practice. After negotiating with the company to start a satellite practice on his own, in late 1980, when he was thirty-one, Acer left Opa-locka. He was remembered by acquaintances there as seeming 'benevolent' and 'humanistic.'"[1]

"Acer seems like he was a nice guy," Artie chimed in.

"That's what people thought who knew him superficially," I responded.

"Did he have any close friends?" Barb queried.

"According to Runnells he had only two—a heterosexual woman named Maureen Englebart who Acer employed as his office manager from the time he opened to the day he closed his dental office (1981-1989) and a homosexual man named Ed Parsons. Though neither one might be considered totally free from bias, it's interesting that the CDC choose to believe Mrs. Englebart, Acer's long time paid employee who according to Runnells:"

> Continued to deny, even under oath, that she knew of his [Acer's] true affliction... According to Acer's parents, Acer had told her in confidence that he had AIDS.[2]

"I find it ironic that the CDC would choose to believe her rather than Parsons," Jackie added.

"Wait, I'm getting lost," admitted Barbara.

"Let me explain," I offered. "Parsons was Acer's best gay friend. The two of them spent a lot of time together discussing the politics of AIDS, and Parsons was the one who fingered Acer for being angry and rebellious against the CDC for losing the war on AIDS. Here, read what Runnells wrote."

I dusted the sand off the cover of *AIDS in the Dental Office?*, opened it to the yellow and pink highlights on page 71, and handed it to Barb.

> The picture painted by Anonym (Runnells's name for Parsons) is that Acer was a troubled, angry alcoholic who, particularly when he drank, displayed his anger against society and the complicated issues surrounding AIDS—the lack of response to the needs for AIDS research, treatment funding by the federal government, the public perception that AIDS is a homosexual disease . . .[3]

"Apparently, Parsons approached Bergalis's attorney Montgomery after seeing Acer's picture in the newspaper and reading that he alleged to being bisexual. Here read this," I grabbed the book from Barbara's hands and turned to an ear-marked page bearing Parsons's testimony:

" I read he was bisexual. There was nothing bisexual about David Acer... Not at all. Absolutely not... and I resent those statements . . ."

"Why would that be?

"It's a falsehood... It's not the truth... We joke about it. Bisexual where? He liked men and boys. Bi what?

I just refuse to feed that (homophobia) wherever it's coming from. I don't want to be part of that.

I think it's probably based on fear. It makes him sort of less of a bad person, I guess. I think with bisexuality I can tell you personally what I believe bi— bisexuality really is for many individuals based on my personal experience meeting people, I think it's conflict, synonymous with conflict . . .

David was very concerned as many of us had been in the past few years about being identified as a homosexual and society's reaction to that...

At that particular point in time one of the conversations we had was the automatic assumption if an individual was homosexual he was HIV infected. That represents, for obvious reasons, a problem."

Here, read this part of his testimony too:"

"What happened was David was angry. He was very anry. I guess he had a right to be. Kimberly Bergalis was very angry, so was the family. That's a natural reaction to a diagnosis like that. But I had a conversation with David that bothered me. It has bothered me for quite a while...

He had been drinking. He—we discussed AIDS again. I think I mentioned a friend of mine had been diagnosed and he discussed with me—he verbalized some opinions and some feelings, and he said something to the effect that, well, our society does not want to address the issue because they perceive it to be a homosexual problem, and when it begins to affect younger people and grandparents, I think is the words he used, he said then maybe society will do something. I kind of just blew it away. I didn't think much of it...

There was sort of anger there about HIV and what our government was—we got into many, many political discussions where HIV came from, the World Health Organization theory and all of these various conversations about it...

And then ultimately after Kim's death there was just something that bothered me about the last conversation I had with him, about this disease infecting other main stream people that just had not set well with me. So we got to get to the truth."

Barbara handed the book back to me.

I went on. "Parsons was then asked on cross examination,

"Are you saying that you interpreted that comment to mean that you felt Dr. Acer was potentially deliberately infecting his patients?"

"He answered:"

" I think so. We had—as I said, we had numerous conversations about AIDS and politics and trans-mission. What he said was when HIV begins to affect main stream—I think the word he used was main stream America, when we start seeing people who are—I think the word he used was adolescents and grandmothers, then maybe something will be done, something to that effect."

"Pretty intense," Barbara acknowledged.

"According to Runnells," I continued, "Parson's tes-timony could not be trusted because investigators felt he had a personal agenda for reporting what he did about Acer. Parsons was suspected of attempting to further the homosexual/gay rights cause by implicating Acer in an attempt to bring the issue of AIDS to the American main-stream.[4] It will be extremely ironic if Acer is proven to be a killer, and Parsons was right. In trusting Acer's family and his other superficial heterosexual acquaintances, the CDC officials will have brought more harm upon them-selves and the image of the CDC than the gay rights move-ment could ever bring."

Jackie kept the ball rolling, "Runnells also reported that prior to making any major business or career deci-sions, Acer would always consult his mother." She reached for Runnells's book and opened it to one of sev-eral pages I had marked with a paperclip, and cited the highlighted text:

Although Harriett was very much a part of helping David locate his practice... and in helping him get started, later she was to say: "I assisted him in no way. He chose it and then began furnishing his office"...Although Harriett refused credit, she helped David choose attractive and functional furnishings...[1]

"In her eyes," Runnells recorded,

David was very much on his own. David was not a 'mama's boy.' She bristled at any suggestion that her eldest son was not completely independent. In fact, she was extremely protective of David and he, in turn, was the same with her.[1]

The Psychologist Smells Trouble

There is clearly a tremendous conflict here, I thought. "Barbara, let me ask you this—how can a mother who is *extremely protective* of her son, involved in every major decision he makes, defensively claim that he operates *completely independent* of her?"

"You're right Len. That doesn't seem right to me either."

"A neurolinguistic programming therapist might say that Harriett Acer's words do not match her physiology and emotions. A keen psychologist might suspect there is denial and repressed conflict operating, while a behavioral scientist would claim there is cognitive behavioral dissonance or belief-behavioral inconsistency," I argued.

"Another observation," Jackie pointed out, "is that David was clearly unlike other young men. Runnells revealed later in his book that, despite denying it to investigators and hiding it from his parents and heterosexual acquaintances, Acer's preference was for "men and boys." If he contracted hepatitis B infection sexually at age twenty, it is likely that by 1989 he had been actively involved in gay sex for nearly two decades. He probably realized that he was homosexual even longer than this given the fact that homosexuality is a genetic as well as a learned (behavioral/developmental) trait."

"All this time he hid this information from his mother probably thinking it would kill her to know the truth," I added then continued, "It seems to me that Harriett, on the other hand, lived in denial. 'What! Not my son. He's no mama's boy.' That her son was somehow different, effeminate, or less than adequate in her eyes would have been very hard for her to accept."

"I've got it here," Jackie interrupted. "Runnells writes,"

One can only imagine how difficult it was for Acer's parents to make the transition from a Midwest family with roots in the depression era when homosexuality was often considered a 'sin against God' to the modern era of accepting.[5]

"Runnells also observed that Harriett 'bristled at any suggestion that her eldest son was not completely... (anything),'[1] which demonstrates to me her defensiveness as well as her denial. Such a response pattern would indicate that Harriett actually felt extremely insecure about David," I argued. "People only become *extremely protective* when they feel the one they're protecting is vulnerable, likely to be attacked or harmed somehow. Likewise, people only get defensive when they feel vulnerable, attacked, or insecure themselves. In other words, Mrs. Acer was most likely afraid that David needed her help to survive and/or thrive."

"Yeah, but you could argue that it would be natural for David to feel protective of his mother. She was, after all, his primary caregiver and model during childhood.

The fact that his father passed away when he was young probably brought him closer to Harriett, encouraging their interdependence," Barbara reasoned.

"That may be true," I responded to Barb's challenge, "But is it possible that *extreme* protectionism could have resulted merely from the loss of his father. This type of behavior, which Runnells reports, was in effect since early childhood, would have required David, at an early age, to also have felt that his mother was somehow extremely vulnerable, attacked, or defenseless. The picture this knowledge invites in my mind is one of possible abuse."

"That possible, Len," Barb admitted, "Could it be that David and his mother were both abused, assaulted, or threatened by the same individual, perhaps even at the same time?"

"That would account for their compulsion towards extreme mutual protectionism wouldn't it?"

"The most traumatic possibility would have been sexual assault, but it could have been some other physical/emotional abuse as well."

"That would support the observation of a life-long pattern of extreme mutual protectionism."

"And since Acer had relied on Harriett to help him make most major life decisions, it would naturally make him feel extremely vulnerable if she were threatened in any way," Barbara added, "This pattern likely started with the death of his father and continued throughout his life."

"Unfortunately for David, however," Jackie contributed, "at a time when he was grieving over his father's death, his mother probably needed to give her greater attention to his younger brother. I can totally relate to the effort required, from our experience with Alena. Young kids demand a lot of attention. This relationship probably left David feeling unattended, or even completely left out."

"Good point," I said. "To explain David's adult behaviors, you must look to his childhood. Acer's adult pattern of introversion and isolation, which was commonly observed by just about everyone who knew him including his parents, must have begun when he was a child. Emotions and behaviors that are reinforced consistently enough in childhood generate the same conditions throughout life. That seems to fit the Acer profile."

The Troubled Side of Dr. David Acer

"Let's continue," I said as I shuffled the deck for the next card.

"During the 1980s, Acer maintained at least two distinct and conflicting personas. One was a quiet and gentle loner; the other was a loud, aggressive, and gay sex fanatic. As documented by Runnells,"

> He was two beings, living two carefully separated and diametrically opposed lives.[6]

"Wow, a real Jekyll and Hyde type," Artie observed.

"That's exactly what Bob Runnells called him," I replied.

"According to his heterosexual acquaintances, Acer was essentially unremarkable: laid-back, intelligent, technically competent, reclusive, introverted, quiet, and even shy. Good friends, Maureen Englebart, and her husband Richard, his tennis and after-match drinking partner, knew the man to be very kind, gentle, and never having 'a bad word to say about anybody.'⁷ He was generally accepted by his patients, at least until his physical appearance and emotional state began to reveal that he had AIDS."

I turned to the next card and said, "Here's my summary of Acer's most commonly observed positive and negative personality traits." I read out loud the list of adjectives I had documented (see Table 2.)

A History of Deceit

"The first knowledge that Acer might be infected with the AIDS virus came from a former sex partner who contacted Acer during the summer of 1985. He discussed his HIV infection and encouraged Acer to go for testing. Acer refused. It was shortly thereafter that Acer met Edward Parsons and the two became relatively close friends," I shared. "About a year later, in July and August 1986, Acer began to experience chronic fatigue, intermittent fevers, and diarrhea. On self-examination he discovered that the lymph nodes under his right armpit were swollen and sore. Thinking that it might be the beginning of AIDS, and not wanting to let word of his lifestyle or illness leak out in his community, he decided to drive a couple of hours south to Ft. Lauderdale to be tested at a laboratory called MedPath. The test came back positive, and Paul Besong, the technician, encouraged Acer to see a local physician, Dr. Frank Gutierrez. Gutierrez, according to Besong and documented by Runnells, was 'known

for his competent and sympathetic counseling of infected persons.'"[7]

"Isn't that what you're working on too?" Barbara
asked.

"Yup. That he was able to go to an independent testing lab and get tested without the slightest bit of counseling first is a crime. I'm sure you can appreciate how
important it is to be counseled before testing and be prepared for a positive test result."

I flipped to the next card. "On August 27, 1986 Acer
visited Dr. Gutierrez for the first time. Using his alias,
David 'Johnson,' he informed Gutierrez that Medpath
had referred him for HIV counseling and care. He did not
disclose the fact that he was a dentist, nor a homosexual,
nor even his military service record. Acer reported that
his last medical examination was two years earlier, that
he was unmarried, and that his last sexual contact was
'two months ago and he did not use a condom.' He also
informed Gutierrez that he became infected with hepatitis B in 1969, had two bouts of inflammation in his ure-
thra, and suffered a recurring lesion on his penis."

"Sounds like a classic STD case," Barbara concluded.

"According to Runnells, and I quote:"

' Johnson's' sexual preference was not discussed.
Gutierrez always made a special effort to not in-
quire into unnecessary personal questions. As a
result, he did not ask 'Johnson' about his sexual
preference. He addressed only the medical questions he determined were necessary to provide
state-of-the-art HIV counseling.[7]

"State-of-the-art?" Barbara exclaimed with a contemptuous look on her face. "Give me a break. The guy fails to discuss sexual preferences, sexual behaviors, and the patient's emotional stability and concerns—and he calls that state-of-the-art?"

"Barb, you've got to remember that the standard of care back then was different from what it is today. Today, the standard requires that thorough pre and post-HIV test counseling be done, including assessing the patient's emotional readiness for the bad news," I retorted. "But back then, the standards were not so clear. Even today, despite a clear counseling protocol developed and promoted by public health departments, most physicians don't do what's recommended to avert the risks to test subjects and the public from the HIV-positive person being emotionally unprepared and unstable at the time of the test.

"Still," Barb defended, "In Acer's case, thorough counseling could have averted the entire affair. Failure to diagnose Acer's emotional instability represented a monumental risk."

"That's true, but lets move on." I flipped to the next card. "Acer returned to Gutierrez again on December 3, 1986. It was during this visit that the doctor probably informed 'Johnson' that he had progressed into the middle stage of HIV infection known as ARC (AIDS Related Complex.) Though not noted in his records, Dr. Gutierrez allegedly reinforced the need for 'Johnson' to practice 'safe sex'[8]."

"I'll bet he really listened," Barbara said sarcastically.

"Unfortunately for many gay men on Florida's east coast, he didn't."

Acer Develops Kaposi's Sarcoma

Following a brief, but refreshing swim in the cold Atlantic waters, our group retrenched for the next round of discussions. I dusted the sand off the notecards and forged ahead.

"Toward the end of August 1987, Acer began to notice a swelling on the palate of his mouth. As a dentist knowledgeable about AIDS, he was likely aware that this was Kaposi's sarcoma (KS), a common oral cancer predominantly found in people with AIDS."

"Isn't it also more predominant in homosexual men with AIDS?" Barbara asked.

"Very good, Barbara. You'll see." I continued, "In order to be sure, on September 16, 1987, he chose to visit a West Palm Beach oral surgeon by the name of Dr. Rolf Wolfrom. Again, Acer used his alias and did not report to Wolfrom the diagnosis of HIV disease established over thirteen months earlier by Gutierrez. He simply asked Wolfrom to biopsy the growth, which he did, removing a three by four millimeter tumor from the roof of Acer's mouth. This tissue sample was sent to Palm Beach Pathology Laboratories for examination and diagnosis. Two days later, a Dr. Hossein Hoghooghi reported to Wolfrom that he could not make a definite diagnosis. According to Wolfrom, Hoghooghi suspected KS, but wanted to know more about the patient's personal lifestyle as this form of cancer in the United States is rare and primarily affects homosexual men."

"Ah. that's what I thought."

"So Wolfrom telephoned 'Johnson' to learn more about his personal and sexual history. The ensuing conversations and events were documented by Runnells:"

On September 21st Wolfrom called Acer and relayed that...the pathologist was interested in whether or not there was any homosexual activity in his past, and he did [finally] admit to that ...over the phone. On the 23rd Wolfrom recorded: Patient admits to being homosexual... He has been informed one and one half years ago that he was advised of being exposed to the AIDS virus... During this time he had regular physical exams by Dr. Frank Gutierrez in Fort Lauderdale with no ARC/AIDS symptoms.[9]

" Runnells pointed out that this last statement was another lie."

"Another frank expression of Acer's denial," Jackie added.

"Or both," Barbara said.

Acer's Case and True Identity Get Reported

"You know it's standard practice for physicians and surgeons, upon diagnosing a patient with AIDS, to contact public health authorities to register the case," I explained to Barb and Artie. "State and local public health departments are then responsible for relaying this information to the CDC. According to legal testimony, Wolfrom immediately followed this protocol and contacted the PBCPHU to identify 'Johnson' and report his case of AIDS. However, at this point, he was still unaware that Acer was a dentist practicing in Jensen Beach."

"According to Runnells's investigation," I continued, "over the next few days, while awaiting the receipt of additional laboratory information about 'Johnson's' cancer, a concerned Wolfrom repeatedly talked with 'Johnson' about his case. During these discussions, Acer finally admitted to Wolfrom that he was a practicing dentist. With this information, Wolfrom expressed his concern about the possibility of Acer passing his infection on to patients. He said to Acer," I looked down at my notecard and read:

" In my opinion it seems that the safest thing to do would be to stop practicing and not to continue to practice."

"Acer's response was not what Wolfrom expected or wanted to hear. He simply denied any threat to patients and stated that he always wore gloves, implying that he would continue to see patients."[10]

"That's when Wolfrom, disturbed by Acer's attitude and comments, decided to phone his attorney for legal advice," Jackie added. Alena was now nursing quietly—allowing Jackie to join the conversation. "His personal attorney then told him to notify the authorities at once."

"So Wolfrom called the health department again?" Barb queried.

"Right," I answered. "This time to inform them about Acer's true identity as a dentist practicing in Jensen Beach. He most likely also reported the potentially lethal dentist to the Florida State Dental Board to see what, if anything, they could do to prevent Acer from practicing and passing the AIDS virus on to his patients."

"Unfortunately," I explained, "though the HRS investigators undoubtedly relayed Wolfrom's complaint and AIDS case report through legal channels, most likely referring him to report Acer to the state dental board, few precedents had been established for public health or licensing agencies to deal effectively with health care workers suffering from AIDS. The laws in most states at the time were ambiguous and/or favored uncompromised patient and professional rights to confidentiality. Even today 'duty to warn' and 'patient notification' laws are non-existent in many states or are still being contested in courtrooms throughout the country. What happened in the Acer case, however, hopefully will never happen again—Acer was allowed to practice without the least supervision by medical or mental health personnel."

Acer's Deadly Activities Continue

"Following the diagnosis of oral cancer and AIDS, Acer managed to hold himself together well enough to continue practicing for more than two years," Artie and Barb listened intently and Jackie smiled down at our nursing angel.

"During the more than three years between Acer's ARC diagnosis and the time he stopped practicing, according to CDC investigators, his medical records never indicated any bleeding disorders, hand dermatitis, hand injuries, or dementia. No indication of nerve problems or shakiness was present, although no detailed neurologic examination or testing was recorded in his medical records.[11] This means either that his medical records were ineptly kept, which is questionable, considering that besides Gutierrez, he had visited several other reputable health professionals and institutions including Miami's V.A. Hospital and the V.A. Ambulatory Care Clinic in Riviera Beach. Could they all have missed diagnosing these generally obvious conditions, or was Acer able to remain free of these signs and symptoms?" I queried the group.

"Maybe he didn't report these problems when they examined him and asked him his chief complaints and medical history," Barbara added.

Jackie perked up, "Acer was very skilled at projecting the image he wanted people to accept.[3] If he had no outward signs of AIDS, then he could have easily persuaded his few friends, family, patients, and dental staff members that he was not sick."

"That's apparently what happened," I interjected. "Runnells reported that Acer even denied his afflictions to his health care professionals." "He could only keep that up for so long. By the Spring of 1989, Acer's death cloak began to show. Always proud of his looks, he began to lose his hair and healthy appearance. It was during this stage of his illness that an employee of the Martin County Public Defender's Office, visited him for treatment and was spooked by his ghostly appearance and personality," Jackie contributed as she lay a sleeping Alena softly down on the shady part of our blanket.

"But despite his weight loss and ghostly appearance," I interrupted, "he continued to solicit gay men and naive boys for sex during his frequent outings to homosexual bars and night clubs... Jack, let me see the book."

Jackie handed me *AIDS in the Dental Office?* and I flipped the earmarked pages till I found what I was looking for. "Here, Runnells documents Acer's disrespect for human life this way:"

> At the same time that Acer was regularly visiting Gutierrez to track progress of his disease and even after being told that he had AIDS, he continued to pursue his lifestyle without telling partners that he was infected. The record indicates that he aggressively sought to satisfy his sexual desires until his health reached a point where he was no longer physically able to continue... In one instance, after recognizing a picture of Acer in a newspaper, one gay individual contacted Kimberly's attorneys to describe how Acer had propositioned him to have sex. The individual was also HIV-positive and, after a short conversation with David, suspected that Acer had AIDS. The individual volunteered his testimony because he felt that Acer's behavior was negligent and that Acer was purposely hiding his infection, thereby placing other gays at risk through his selfish and irresponsible lifestyle. He felt that, because Acer was irresponsible in his sexual lifestyle, he was probably irresponsible in his dental practice and that the irresponsibility may have led to Kim's and the other patients' infections.[9]

"That's incredible," Artie acknowledged. "The guy had to be a real loon."

"A very *smart* and *devious* loon," I stressed.

A Psychoanalytic Interpretation of Acer's "Mainstream" Intent

"Barbara, will you tell me this—what is the difference between exposing dental patients to lethal injections of HIV tainted blood and indiscriminately injecting HIV infected sperm into unsuspecting gays' bodies?"

"The former lacks the hedonistic intent of the latter," Barb answered.

"But assures that Acer's place in health care history would be reserved," Jackie added.

"Let's look at Acer from a psychoanalytic perspective," I challenged the group. "According to Runnells, Acer was a closet bisexual, unwilling to admit to being a homosexual—as though the difference between bisexuality and homosexuality was spiritually vast. Why, besides not wanting his mother to find out, do you think that he wouldn't admit to being a homosexual?"

"Maybe he saw himself as a bridge between both worlds. His plan then would be motivated to bring mainstream America and the gay community into the same battle against AIDS. Parsons's testimony appears to support this theory," Jackie advanced.

"Maybe he defended his bisexuality as an attempt to distance himself from and thus defend the gay community from the negative publicity the case would bring. Perhaps Kimberly Bergalis becoming so quickly caught him by surprise. He may have expected to be dead by the time his victims were identified. Then these issues of sexuality would have been buried along with him, leaving investigators even more confused," I speculated.

"That sounds like a likely scenario," Barb conceded.

"In any case," I continued, "Acer maintained this elite—though disputed—description of himself to the very end. The fact that he would go down in history as being the 'gay' dentist who infected so many patients would ironically add additional social stigma to the gay community."

As she reached for the cooler and began to pour refreshments for the thirsty crew, Jackie reasoned, "You know people will question these psychosocial theories about Acer's intent. They'll argue, like Runnells, that Acer wouldn't openly admit to being a homosexual because of the loss this might bring to his dental practice in the conservative suburb of Stuart."

"Jack, I told you before, psychopathology reaches much deeper than such superficial explanations. It is very clear—Acer never came to embrace his own homosexuality—he hid it as though ashamed, guilty, or socially vulnerable. People who reject certain parts of themselves, for whatever reason, commonly project their loss of self-esteem onto others; they see others as inferior and/or dangerous. If they wholeheartedly accepted people in their social circles, they would also have to come to terms with that irritating part of themselves. The process of revealing one's unique self is often very painful, and not many travel the difficult path to self-discovery."

"This would explain why Acer disrespected the lives of homosexuals and withdrew from heterosexuals," Barbara picked up quickly on my idea.

"Precisely Barb. Acer was clearly hung-up about being gay. He successfully hid his homosexuality from his patients and professional acquaintances, and most urgently, he never wanted to let his parents, *especially his mother,* know he was less than what they imagined. Acer's stepfather testified that David kept his homosexuality and illness very much a secret. Runnells quoted Victor Acer as saying:"

" After we found out about it, he said he had hoped that they would be able to find a vaccine or a cure or something so he could get cured without our ever having to know that he had AIDS."[12]

"He also failed to support gay rights organizations and would not attend their demonstrations," Jackie pointed out. "Even after he had developed AIDS, he refused to join his homosexual friends in their fight against homophobia, allegedly because he was afraid his patients, family and heterosexual acquaintances would learn he was gay. He probably felt somewhat torn and guilty about that too."

"It seems he was stuck in the middle of both gay and straight worlds," Barbara reasoned.

"That's how it appears to me. His greatest death bed challenge was to explain to his mother how he became exposed. Only at the very end was he able to admit his sexual preference to her. One of his brothers sent Harriett Acer *How Will I Tell My Mother,* a book Acer's social worker hoped would help Acer inform his extremely protective mother that her son had been living a dual life, and his homosexuality was responsible for his AIDS. Acer kept this knowledge from everyone until his final days. Even then, he was unable to express or discuss his conflicting emotions."[5]

"He also kept the deadly-aggressive side of himself, well hidden," Jackie mentioned. "Edward Parsons frequently witnessed both Acer personalities and knew the dangerous side of him most intimately."

"Who's Parsons again?" queried Artie.

"Parsons was Acer's best gay friend, some believe they were lovers. Anyway, he was a male nurse who shared Acer's medical knowledge, political views, sexual preferences, and terminal illness. They were as close as Acer's defenses probably would allow."

"The most important thing about Parsons was that he and his testimony were overlooked by the CDC and HRS investigators. He had revealed to Robert Montgomery, Bergalis's attorney, during sworn testimony that Acer would commonly go from being a very kind and gentle man to an inebriated alcoholic who drank until he was sloppy and aggressive. In this state, Parsons explained, he would be able to come on to men and boys a lot more.[13] The public health investigators along with the Florida attorney general's office just decided to overlook Parson's testimony."

I drew the next notecard which read: "In June of 1989, Acer confirmed his history of alcoholism with Mildred Gelfand, a licensed social worker and counselor, who documented according to Runnells, a 'history of excessive drinking prior to diagnosis [with AIDS, and] no drinking since.' Acer's claim of sobriety, however was later disputed by Parsons as well as another gay acquaintance who stated he continued to drink to help him satisfy his sexual compulsions, even after he knew he had AIDS and that he was a threat to others."[14]

"Notice," I said to the group, "there's at least two people Runnells cites as having said negative things about Acer compared with none reported by the CDC. According to these people, Acer was a consistent liar, very secretive and potentially very deadly. He never admitted he had AIDS and never warned the numerous unsuspecting gay men and boys he lured into sex. Acer himself reported to his physician as many as *150 sex partners over a ten-year period, and he was most likely lying on the conservative side so as not to raise a red flag.*"[14]

"It's interesting that the CDC report also said nothing about Acer's sexual promiscuity. They did report interviewing all of Acer's health care professionals, so surely they would have noted how much sex he was having, and that there was an imbalance there."

"It's equally suspicious they neglected to report anything about his alcoholism," Jackie observed.

"You bet it is," I responded as I got up to stretch my legs. "The whole thing smacks of a cover-up."

Chapter 9.
A Mission of
Homicide and Suicide

We spent the rest of the holiday weekend relaxing and discussing the Acer case with our friends, and after they left, I settled back to analyze Acer's history in greater detail.

I first considered how people tend to withdraw and become reclusive as a result of feeling—or actually being—traumatized, abused, persecuted, neglected, and/or attacked during early childhood by parents or significant others.

The fact that David Acer was described as a very kind and sensitive recluse by some people, and aggressive and sloppy by others would indicate that the successful dentist might have been suffering from what some psychoanalysts call an affective (depressive) disorder, I thought.

I decided to research the prevalence of depression and chemical dependency among dentists and found that both are common among dentists as well as the general public. One article noted that "dentists tend to be highly stressed perfectionists" who tend towards chemical dependency—alcohol being the most commonly abused drug of choice.[1] Approximately 15 percent of dentists maintain a chemical dependency while between 16 and 20 percent of the general population suffers depressive symptoms, alcoholism being one.

Interesting but nothing particularly unusual, I thought.

My literature search also taught me that a variety of risk factors are strongly associated with affective (depressive) disorders including: stressful life events, genetic predisposition, personal vulnerability to stress based on personality and social learning, and biological abnormalities which may be acquired after birth or inherited.[2]

With the growing evidence of genetic transmission of depressive disorders, one reputable study concluded that individuals have a twenty times greater chance of suffering a depressive disorder if a parent or child maintained this illness.[3]

If only I knew more about Harriett Acer, I thought. *Maybe then I could understand David better.* So despite having heard that she and her family had been closed to such inquiries, I attempted to contact her.

Harriett and Victor, I soon learned, maintained an unlisted telephone number. David's stepbrother Kenneth however, also lived in the Pittsburgh area, and I was able to get his number and answering machine on the first try.

After not having my message returned, I called again the following morning. This time Kenneth answered and after explaining very diplomatically who I was and why I wanted to speak with his mother, Kenneth made it quite clear that the Acer family had no intention of discussing David's case any further.

"It's nice to know that so many people are so interested in David, but the family does not wish to discuss it any more," Kenneth said.

"Sure. I understand. It must be very difficult for all of you," I sympathized. "Well, I won't bother you again."

I sat back to reflect. *I can't let this throw me.* I affirmed. *I can't give up just because the family won't reveal their secrets.* Then I resumed my search for meaning in the information Runnells had published.

That night, Jackie and I joined forces again to review the known facts. "Being gay—a result of both genetics and social learning—and given the prevalence of homophobia, Acer would naturally have felt somehow different and probably even inferior during his childhood and adolescence," I established. "His difference would have made it much more difficult for him to bond with any straight male model. If this were the case, any parental neglect or psychological deprivation would have led the young Acer to close down his sense of feeling or emotional response as he would not have been able to reach out to a bonded model or peer."[4]

Jackie added, "this could have helped to establish the introverted behavior Runnells documented and would also help to explain why another one of Acer's heterosexual friends said he, 'never had a bad word to say about anyone.'"[5]

"With a diminished emotional response plus his tendency towards quiet isolation, Acer would not be likely to have expressed negative emotions or attitudes towards others. People who bear their own weighty cross, as Acer was undoubtedly forced to do in a world which wouldn't accept his gayness, are far less inclined to criticize others who may have established secure personal identities. That's the essential challenge for gays developing in homophobic societies."

Then it occurred to both of us that society must also be considered at least partially accountable for sealing Acer's fate along with the fate of the many men and boys he could have infected and the patients whom we believed he selectively infected.

AIDS, Depression and Suicide

I also reviewed the scientific literature on AIDS, depression and suicide, as it occurred to me that *Acer, a chronic drinker, might have been suicidal as well.* I recalled from my post-doctorate training that heavy drinking had been shown to be a prolonged form of suicide.[6] *Maybe Acer maintained a conscious and/or subconscious death wish.*

Finally it struck me, *the part of Acer—his gay identity, which he worked so hard to hide—would soon be revealed by AIDS. This must have been a great source of anxiety for him.*

Then I read two other review articles[7,8] which showed the most common predictors of suicide are alcohol abuse, anxiety, depression, and aggressive behavior. *Acer had displayed all of these,* I realized.

Other studies I read also showed that among these correlates or predictors of suicidal thoughts, plans, and attempts, the two most consistently related to self-destruction are aggressive/compulsive behavior and alcohol use.[8] Science proved the combination of negative life events, low self-esteem, and substance abuse increased the risk of serious depression many times.[9]

I also read that among suicidal persons, violent and aggressive outbursts as well as withdrawal and depression were common symptoms.[10] High rates of suicidal behavior had also been observed among juveniles with a history of violent crimes and aggressive behaviors.[11-13] Of these four behaviors, namely violence, aggressive outbursts, withdrawal, and depression, Acer's violence was the only one not observed by friends or family because he did this covertly.

It suddenly became clear to me that Acer was committing suicide on all levels of his being. He was dying of AIDS, a disease of the body's defense system, in which the cells specialized to differentiate between self and non-self were being overwhelmed. *What better metaphor could there be for Acer's unsuccessful struggle to heal his own personal identity crisis,* I thought.

The slow, silent, and purposeful form of suicide that Acer committed through chronic isolation and alcoholism fulfilled a destiny that he and his social environment had created. Then it occurred to me—*the whole, intact Acer had been killed off long ago by a society steeped in bigotry and parents who apparently denied him his innate homosexuality.*

Incapable of accepting his gay self or any other self for that matter, it's only natural that he would turn his mindless aggression toward other gays and, in the end, toward society as a whole.

I was aware of numerous studies which showed chronic use of alcohol to be as destructive to self and society as more obvious and immediate acts like suicide and murder.[6,14] A mountain of publications had documented the link between heavy or frequent alcohol use and negative life events, anxiety, depressive symptoms, lack of social support and low self-esteem.[9,14]

I again brought out the list of adjectives witnesses had used to describe Acer (see Table 1) and dwelled upon the fact that denial, repression, avoidance, isolation, self-reliance (except for maternal dependence), self-interest, self-abuse, anger, aggression, rebelliousness, lying, depression, and alcoholism were all among the negative personality traits and behaviors observed in Acer.

Finally, I reviewed studies which showed that anxiety in gay men infected with HIV is directly related to their level of sexual activity. Studies showed that those with the greatest anxiety were found more likely to practice unsafe sex increasing the risk of transmitting their disease.[15, 16] *If Acer was anxious however, he did not reveal it,* I realized. *Therefore, he probably repressed it. As anxiety and depression are often prominent symptoms of an affective disorder, this would help to explain Acer's compulsive urge for alcohol and sex. His drunken and aggressive attempts at luring other men and boys to have sex with him, which according to observers was his homosexual ritual, were an ineffective and short-lived means of transmuting his repressed feelings and inner conflict.*

Acer's Self Care Regimen

The next morning during our usual hike through the woods, I brought Jackie up to date on what I had learned from my review of the scientific literature relating to anxiety, depression, and suicide among those who carry the AIDS virus. Once up to date, Jackie asked, "All right. What else do we know about Acer that would prove he was a murderer?"

"His medical records," I replied.

"What about them?"

"They show that he would surgically remove cancerous growths from his own mouth using an electro-surg unit."

"What does that prove?"

"To do this he would have had to use anesthetic on himself. Otherwise, he would have felt intense pain as the electrical probe burned through the tissues of his palate. Imagine using cautery to remove tumors growing in your own mouth?" I said.

"That's a grotesque thought," Jackie responded. "But you did a fair amount of restorative dentistry on yourself."

"It's one thing to do a small filling on yourself, but somehow the thought of self administered oral cancer surgery leaves me cold. Acer must have been freaking out."

"I see your point. It does suggest that he brought home and used on himself the anesthetic cartridges, needles and syringe—the homicidal implements required to infect the others," Jackie concluded.

"Right. Though first recorded in his medical records in May of 1989, it is very likely he began his surgical self-care regimen the first week of October, 1987, directly following his initial diagnosis of Kaposi's sarcoma," I speculated.

"Why then?"

"This was the first time that AIDS began distorting his previously unscathed body—violating his intact body image," I replied. "It must have driven him crazy; he was paranoid about his physical appearance."

"That's true. I remember Runnells reported that Acer, was always concerned about his looks."[17]

"Right again. Remember he said that when Acer's hair began to thin, he immediately underwent hair transplants? Looking good was probably vital to satisfying his compulsive sex drive in the gay community."

I continued, "Can you imagine how he felt when this ugly brown cancerous mass began taking over the roof of his mouth? He immediately did what any red-blooded, obsessive/compulsive, AIDS stricken, young American dentist would do--rush down to the dental office to get the electrosurgery unit for home use.

"It's probably no coincidence then, that this date, October 5, 1987— when 'Johnson' learns he has cancer and days later reveals his true identity--was just about ten weeks before he infected Bergalis," Jackie said.

"You got it," I responded, "In his zeal to discharge the intense anger and anxiety built up by his diagnosis, he probably planned the whole affair. Then came the fatal day—December 17, 1987—the day he set his deadly exposures plan into action; the day he removed Kimberly Bergalis's wisdom teeth.

Did you know that Barbara Webb, his second victim, was also in his dental office that day?"

"No," Jackie replied with a look of amazement.

"Yes. I got that from reviewing the CDC report. But he apparently only marked her as a target that day. The grandmother's injection would come later," I said.

"It makes sense," Jackie continued, "that following his diagnosis of KS, Acer would have realized that his days on earth were numbered. He could no longer live in denial. He had nothing to lose now, and only a personal vendetta to resolve."

Denial and Rationalization

The more we talked about it the more sense it made. By serial killing dental patients as Parson's alleged, Acer had more to gain than revenge against the American mainstream. He apparently intended to force the CDC and all of health care into a quandary. Through his eyes it was a brilliant scheme to involve the HRS, CDC, and society as a whole in his struggle with AIDS and homosexuality. His deliberate injecting of selected patients with his blood could easily be interpreted as the expression of aggression he was known to be harboring. Homicidal behavior was at this point well within reason for Acer in his self and social hostile mood.

"To be a serial killer," Jackie theorized as we walked through the woods, "Acer would really have had to be living in denial—lacking any empathy for his victims."

"That's exactly how he lived," I responded. "Acer's denial was a way of life. He shared with stepfather Victor before he died that he had hoped a vaccine or cure for AIDS would have been found early enough to save his life..."

"And save him from having to tell his mother he was gay and dying from the 'gay plague'," Jackie interrupted. "Being so protective of her he probably felt tremendously guilty knowing how much this knowledge would hurt her."

"There's at least one powerful reason he sought re-venge against the CDC-- for not discovering a cure for his AIDS, to save him from being disgraced in the eyes of his mother."

"Look Alena. See the doggie? What does the doggie say?"

"Voff, voff, voff," Alena barked softly.

I continued, "Acer's pattern of denial could also be seen in his denying his gay identity, denying he should be tested, denying he had AIDS, and denying he would succumb to the disease.

As we returned from our walk, we marveled at his plan to get even with a homophobic society and a grossly insensitive health care establishment by infecting the American mainstream, the young and the old, and in such a way as to burden the entire health care system and its principal public health institution, the CDC with an unsolvable mystery. But there was more to Acer's ho-micidal motive that we would soon discover.

The Doubting Thomas

"You know," Jackie said as we entered the house and prepared to get Alena out of the backpack, "there are many people who will challenge you on this investiga-tion into Acer's forensic psychology. Runnells, for ex-ample, believes that Acer wouldn't have intentionally infected his patients, fearing the attention an investiga-tion might have brought him and his successful dental practice. Surely, a man who desperately desired isola-tion and wanted to keep his dental practice intact would not be so inclined, Runnells argued."[18]

"You're right, Jack, but Runnells didn't have the behavioral science background to evaluate Acer's apparent psychopathology. Runnells's explanation is too superficial. Psychopathology runs deep. A deeply repressed part of Acer was literally dying for his sexual orientation to be revealed. Revealing his true identity was ultimately the only way in which he could be healed of all his symptoms: his emotional disorder, his depressive symptoms, his alcoholism, and his aggression which were all due to him burying his true feelings, homosexuality, and personality for so long. It's natural that when he foresaw the end of his life he would act violently to discharge the repressed tension and anxiety he had been holding back since childhood."

"Do you think she needs a diaper change?"

I followed Jackie into the nursery and continued. "To help ease his pain, Acer withdrew to become the quiet recluse everyone who knew him observed. The chronic play between isolation and aggression is a depressive syndrome which borders on mania. Suicide, the ultimate form of isolation, Acer committed slowly."

"Aggression and revenge against those he targeted—his victims, the CDC, organized health care, and society as a whole—would follow even after his demise."

"Brilliant for a demented and tormented man."

"But the doubting Thomas may ask why would Acer intend to destroy the most revered accomplishment of his life before killing himself?" Jackie charged.

"This fits with his pattern of self-abuse," I defended. "Don't you see? For someone steeped in denial, anger, guilt, and self, and social aggression it is logical that Acer would, at least on a subconscious level, impulsively destroy the most meaningful thing in his life—his dental career."

"Maybe he also didn't think Bergalis and the others would be discovered so quickly?"

"That's very likely."

Unhappy and Dissatisfied with Self and Society

"Acer was a very unhappy and dissatisfied man," I continued. "Research shows the psychological states of unhappiness and dissatisfaction, as well as isolation and alienation lead to the use of mood-altering drugs such as alcohol.[19,20]

"Why do you think that is?"

"Because of their effects on self-esteem and anxiety. Alcohol is very therapeutic for anxiety and low self-esteem. Acer's chronic alcoholism dulled the pain and awareness that he was not what his parents wanted him to be, not who his patients and staff thought he was. He was alone, isolated, angry, and anxious about dying from AIDS. Parsons observed this. Research also shows that anxiety and low self-esteem makes people more likely to risk harm, and motivates people to try to conform to risky peer norms."[21]

"Here hold these." Jackie handed me Alena's diaper clips. "What do you mean by conforming to risky peer norms?"

"Consider the fact that Acer tried to fit in, but he didn't fit anywhere. He knew he couldn't fit into straight society because he was innately gay, so he withdrew from the straight world and then condemned it for his pain.

He tried to conform to the standards of the gay community, but that didn't work either. To the extent that cruis-
ing the beaches and indiscriminate sex was a measure of
gay norms, Acer excelled in his effort to conform. To the
degree that being gay meant political activism, Acer was
a subdued failure. This too likely troubled him. The
marches and demonstrations he wouldn't allow himself
to attend were his march to freedom."

"O.K. give me the clips."

"Here."

I continued despite Alena's verbal protest against being laid down.

"Acer's gay acquaintances testified that Acer continued to cruise the gay beach on Hutchinson Island, and
search the bars up and down the Florida coast for one
night stands despite knowledge that he was highly infectious and even very sick with AIDS."

"Clearly, he was very troubled and confused."

"Likewise, despite his disabling illness, he continued
to practice dentistry—allegedly for financial reasons."

"Apparently, even Harold Jaffe admitted Acer was
self-interested and deceitful."

"Where did you hear that?"

"I read it in the June 1991 issue of *AIDS Alert*."[22]

"Did you know a month later, Jaffe told the *New York
Times* that since they were still baffled by the events,
they were considering a criminal investigation?"[23]

"No."

"Yes."

Chapter 10.
Why Did the CDC
and HRS Blunder?

The more Jackie and I thought about it, the more suspicious we became that Butterworth or others at the attorney general's office in Florida, knowing all the facts about this case including details about Acer's alcoholism, chronic lying and deceit, pattern of social isolation alternating with homosexual fetishes and aggression, and at least two plausible motives for killing his patients would note an "absence of supporting evidence" surrounding the case.

"Who's kidding whom?" I said to Jackie.

We considered various explanations for this including: a) there are no intelligent life forms in the Florida attorney general's office, or b) officials in the Florida attorney general's office conspired with HRS and CDC officials to ignore the facts in an effort to defend the state and federal organizations against financial liability and avoid the public and political embarrassment a criminal investigation and scandal might bring to public health officials or other political notables.

Given the likelihood of conspiracy to cover-up the truth, we found it most ironic to read the CDC and GAO reports which alleged that Acer's victims covered-up their sexual practices, drug use habits, and financial motives. In the true spirit of Freudian projection the GAO investigators wrote:

Any HIV-positive patients of the dentist had a clear financial incentive to claim that the dentist had been the source of the infection so that monetary damages could be claimed. (Three patients had received $1 million settlements from the dentist's malpractice carrier and additional settlements from the dental care program that provided the dentist's services.) At the very least, potential for financial gain provided incentives for infected patients to deny other risk factors.[1]

The same may be said about the CDC and HRS's incentives for covering up and/or misinterpreting the information they had that indicated Acer had intentionally infected his patients.

Finally, we struggled to understand why the Florida state attorney general's office, in possession of these data, would not have launched a criminal inquiry.

One warm evening towards the middle of July, as we stood out on our upper deck overlooking the harbor lights, Jackie asked, "Why do you think the CDC and HRS blew the investigation?"

Several reasons came to mind as I took a breath of fresh air. "The most likely one is that the chaos at the CDC and HRS was just what the doctor ordered," I responded. "Essentially all the evidence suggests that Acer consciously manipulated public health investigators to force them and all of health care into a state of confusion."

"You mean by organizing the murders in such a way as to not leave a clue and knowing he had nothing to lose since he would shortly be dead, he only had a demented sense of pleasure to gain?"

"I'd bet on it."

"Me too, I guess," Jackie said as she took a seat on the bench. "Acer easily insulated himself from the investigation by hiring Attorney Sawyer. After that, he was able to enjoy at a safe distance and as much as possible, given his ill health, the dominance, power, control, revenge, confusion and torment he engineered."

My wife is beginning to sound like Perry Mason, I thought as I offered my next comment, "Acer knew that he had successfully avoided HRS and CDC investigators almost two-and-a-half years before they first came to investigate him for the Bergalis case. On or around October 5, 1987, HRS and/or CDC agents investigated Acer as an AIDS case because of Wolfrom's report. After Wolfrom knew Acer had lied about his name and occupation on his medical history, upon the recommendation of his attorney, he informed the authorities about Acer being a potential menace to society. Wolfrom probably also cited Acer's deceitful and illegal behavior. Medical records are, after all, legal documents. Runnells reported that the HRS simply refused to act.

"So here we are again. Why do you think they didn't act?" Jackie queried.

"Well, we've talked about the fear of violating confidentiality and anti-discrimination laws. I'd bet the investigators couldn't have given Acer a slap on the wrist if they wanted to. Acer knew this and probably derived great satisfaction from knowing that they couldn't do a damn thing about him."

"Sure, and the absence of negative consequences following an illegal act reinforces the desire to repeat the activity."

I shook my head. "Where do you get these things?" I asked.

"Acer knew he was protected by confidentiality and informed consent laws. He was a trained health professional who also happened to be gay and have AIDS. He had to know all about the policies of HIV-positive patient care and the related health professional and legal risk management concerns. He was on top of all of it, and he knew he had the upper hand with the HRS and CDC."

"He probably also knew that if he was to be investigated for murder, the credibility of the CDC and HRS would be seriously damaged by the revelation that they did nothing to assure the public's health and safety—despite knowing he was seriously ill. The standard practice for public health departments is to refer such cases and complaints to state dental boards who then are supposed to follow them up. Very likely, that's how Acer probably came to receive instructions for continuing to practice dentistry using masks, gloves, and proper sterilization and disinfection procedures. An infection control authority possibly from the PBCPHU, but more likely from the Florida State dental board, must have counseled him about using universal precautions less than ten weeks before he infected Bergalis and soon thereafter the others."

"How can you be sure?"

"The signs are everywhere," I responded.

Acer's Open Letter to his Patients and America

Knowing that Acer knew he was clearly insulated from prosecution and had gained power and control over HRS and CDC investigators, gave Jackie and I a different perspective than Runnells and the others. This was criti-cal in evaluating the famous open letter Acer had written to his patients.

The Acer letter fiasco began when Dr. Howell of the Florida HRS urged Acer to help the authorities to notify Acer's patients regarding their need for HIV testing. The request apparently gave Acer the idea to publish an open letter to his patients just before he died.

Runnells reported that the CDC investigators had first contacted Sawyer and through her Acer, to help them determine if any other patients, besides Bergalis, in his practice had been infected. Because Acer had either de-stroyed or dispersed all patient rosters, records, and ap-pointment schedules, CDC investigators found it nearly impossible to track down the patients he had placed at risk. After a brief holdout, Acer finally consented to their request. According to Runnells, the idea for the open let-ter came from Acer.[2] Everyone, including Acer, knew that the published letter would be picked up by the national press. The letter clearly reflected Acer's thoughts, moti-vations and intent.

In this letter, Acer cited the CDC's liability and in-volvement in the cross infections six times in only eight paragraphs. As you read the letter you will notice it con-demns the CDC and expresses Acer's vendetta, along with his belief that they can't be trusted, and they let him down.

"This is incredibly consistent with the testimony provided by Parsons," Jackie realized after reading the letter while cradling a screaming Alena for her mid-after-noon feeding.

"It's clear to me that Acer intended this to be his final testimonial in support of his demented plan to have the entire cluster of AIDS cases be an extraordinary embarrassment to the CDC," I said gathering up the books and toys the baby had strewn about the floor. "Do you think that might be why the CDC and HRS chose not to acknowledge Parsons or heed his advice?"

"I'm not sure."

"Looking at it from Acer's point of view, at best his plan would destroy the CDC's credibility, burden its resources, and create an unsolvable mystery which would panic the American mainstream about their vulnerability to AIDS. At worst the letter would encourage people to remember him as an innocent, sensitive, and caring dentist who cared very much about his patients' health. What could he lose?"

I sat on the den floor surrounded by papers and continued my analysis. "Though Runnells speculated that some of the harsh words written here against the CDC may have been Attorney Sawyer's contribution—an effort to position her defense against impending law suits—I'll bet he successfully preyed on her seeking protection and someone to carry out his evil directives."

Alena looked up, gave me a pixie-like grin as I submitted to Jackie, "Most authorities claimed that because Acer was willing to write this letter he was being cooperative. If this was truly the case then the political overtones of the letter would not be so apparent."

The letter which appeared in the *Stewart News* on September 6, 1990, is included here for you to decide the intent:

August 31, 1990.

To My Former Patients:

I am David J. Acer, and I have AIDS. I was formerly a dentist in the Martin County area, and if you were my patient, I ask you to please read this letter.

I am writing you this letter because I am concerned that with the recent news regarding me in the local media, you are afraid that you may have been infected with the disease commonly known as AIDS. I want to try to reassure you that it is unlikely you have been infected with the disease from me, and to urge you to seek the free testing and counseling that is available from your local health department.

First, to reassure you as best I can, I want each of you to understand that when I became aware that I had tested positive for the HIV virus (AIDS), I consulted with medical experts on whether I should continue practicing dentistry. I did not want to expose any of my patients to infection with the virus. The experts advised me that as long as I followed the guidelines promulgated by the Centers for Disease Control ('CDC') for health care providers who were infected with HIV (AIDS), that I could safely continue to practice as a dentist, and that I would not infect my patients. I reviewed the CDC guidelines and strictly adhered to them. Each time the CDC revised its guidelines on how a health care provider or worker could safely prevent the transmission of AIDS to patients, I followed those recommendations religiously. Because I was aware that I had the HIV virus, I was extremely careful in how I practiced dentistry. Because the CDC guidelines stated that an infected health care provider could safely continue to provide health care to patients as long as he consulted with his physician on providing health care and followed the guidelines, I felt I could continue to practice dentistry without risk to my patients. I stopped practicing when I became ill with cancer.

It is with great sorrow and some surprise that I read that I am accused of transmitting the HIV virus (AIDS) to one of my patients. I do not understand how such a thing could have happened, and I do not believe it did happen. There was no puncture or cut incurred by me during the procedure, and I followed the CDC guidelines with this patient in the belief that I would safely prevent the infection of the disease as advised by the Centers for Disease Control. If the Centers for Disease Control had advised me to stop practicing because the guidelines were not safe, I would have immediately done so. However, it was my belief that the Centers for Disease Control would never issue guidelines that would put patients and health care workers at risk in transmitting this disease.

However, you understandably are frightened. For your peace of mind, I suggest that you please contact the local health department for free testing and counseling. This can be done anonymously, or you may explain you were my patient, and would like to be reassured that you have not been infected. If the CDC guidelines are valid, you should not be infected.

For Martin County residents, please contact the Martin County Health Unit for free testing, counseling and education for AIDS. The Martin County Health Unit will be open at 8:00 AM, as of Tuesday September 4, 1990, on weekdays, to receive your inquiries. You may also telephone public health staff trained in AIDS testing and counseling at (407) 221-4030 for information. This phone line is open from 8:00 AM to 5:00 PM everyday, including weekends and holidays. If you are worried and anxious about this disease and possible infection, then please call for an appointment for testing and counseling. It is important to be informed of this disease, so you are aware of the dangers and how it can and cannot be transmitted. As fear of the unknown is hard to deal with, but knowledge of what you fear can at least help you know what action to take, if any.

I am sorry I cannot tell you this face to face, but I am dying of this disease. I am very close to the end. I have been putting my affairs in order and saying good bye to my family. It is my desire to die in private peace and quiet with as much dignity as possible. I am very grateful to those who have helped me through this difficult time. It has been extremely hard on my family and especially on my mother who has cared for me and watched me slip away. For this reason, my mother plans to donate property to an organization dedicated to the care of AIDS patients, because these people need help when they are dying with this disease.

Finally, please try to understand. I am a gentle man, and I would never intentionally expose another to this disease. I have cared for people all my life, and to infect anyone with this disease would be contrary to everything I have stood for. I am sorry if the news story has caused you fear and worry.

Sincerely,

David J. Acer

All Lies? Maybe Not

According to Runnells's study, Acer's letter contained several false details. Jackie and I noted these and some others. We also made two novel observations.

First we considered the lies:

Acer claimed in lines 14-18 that he adhered strictly to CDC guidelines. After interviewing Acer's dental staff, Runnells found that this was far from the truth.[3]

He also claimed in lines 13-14 that "I did not want to expose any of my patients to infection with the virus." Given that he himself states that he did not cut himself, the only plausible explanation for the transmissions was by injection, so we considered this statement to be questionable. Later we discovered additional evidence which proved it was obviously false.

In addition, Acer claimed in lines 12 and 23-26 that he consulted with his physician and medical experts regarding continuing to provide dental care under CDC guidelines. Dr. Runnells states that this claim was false.

To defend his position, Runnells pointed to the fact that Acer was told by Wolfrom, that he was a danger to patients and that he should stop practicing dentistry. If you remember, Acer denied that there was a risk given the fact that he was using gloves and masks, which prompted Wolfrom to phone the PBCPHU.

However, clues suggesting that Acer discussed his HIV status and dental activities with HRS authorities are in at least two other places. The most striking is in the official CDC report of the investigation which stated,

> The dentist was known to the Florida Department of Health and Rehabilitative Services investigator as a previously reported AIDS case.[4]

"It's just unbelievable that the HRS and CDC would not follow up with an inquiry, counseling or supervision, knowing that Acer was a dentist who according to

Wolfrom presented a potential public health risk," Jackie lamented.

I got up again to stretch my legs. "That's just the way they operate, Jack. Any other disease report or complaint that presents a risk to the public they jump on. Not AIDS. It's too political. It's the same as the absurdity of not being able to talk openly about AIDS for fear of intense discrimination."

"But you're sure Acer would have had to have been counseled in the use of universal precautions by someone at the HRS or state dental board," Jackie questioned as Alena began to doze off.

"Absolutely."

"Then if a criminal investigation of this case ever occurs," Jackie continued, "it would be prudent to find out who spoke with Acer and how he responded."

"That would be helpful," I conceded.

In addition to the CDC's report about the HRS's previous knowledge of Acer, another confirmation of their association came from Kimberly Bergalis who wrote a stunning condemnation of Nikki Economu and others at the HRS in one of the most intense and heart wrenching letters I ever read. Her letter may be found in its entirety in *AIDS in the Dental Office?* on pages 173-175. Here is one related excerpt:

> Who do I blame?... I blame Dr. Acer and every
> single one of you bastards. Anyone that knew Dr.
> Acer was infected and had full-blown AIDS and
> stood by not doing a damn thing about it. You are
> all just as guilty as he was. You've ruined my life
> and my family's. I forgive Dr. Acer because I believe

the disease affected his mind. He wasn't able to think properly and he continued to practice.... but I have a harder time forgiving your organization [the HRS/CDC].[5]

"Would you spread Alena's blanket out so I can put her down to sleep?"

I laid the patchwork quilt down and patted it flat.

"Ironically, the only thing Kimberly Bergalis and David Acer had in common was their mutual contempt for the HRS and CDC," I said.

"Perhaps what moved Kimberly to become the staunch crusader for full HIV disclosure in health care was the intense suffering she endured from the HRS and CDC's attempt to blame her and their negligence in allowing Acer to continue practicing unsupervised," Jackie theorized.

"You know what still troubles me?"

"What?" Jackie responded as she laid Alena down to sleep.

"Well Acer informed Wolfrom that he had been seeing Dr. Gutierrez in Ft. Lauderdale for medical care. Wolfrom even wrote this in Acer's records. When Wolfrom informed the HRS and possibly the Florida State Dental Board about Acer's case, he must have informed them about Dr. Gutierrez because he was very concerned about Acer's health and competence right?"

"Right."

"He probably also informed the authorities that Acer had used an alias. In any case, had the HRS simply responded to Wolfrom's concerns or reviewed his or

Gutierrez's records when they initially investigated Acer as an AIDS case, they would have found he had been lying about his name and occupation, a symptom of his insecurity and emotional instability."

"Or, they may have discovered he was unstable, and for whatever reason—possibly legal related to informed consent laws—chose not to do anything about it."

"Yeah, but Acer was a pretty smooth talker with a deceptive disposition even though inside he was a time bomb set to go off... Do you want some juice or water?"

"Sure."

As I walked into the kitchen for refreshments, the Wolfrom episode raced through my head: *Acer's case investigator and/or his infection control counselor, whose identity was being withheld by the authorities, had to have been very close to discovering that Acer was a chronic liar, not to be trusted at all—a finding which could have saved them, the CDC, Acer's victims and the American public all the fears and misfortunes his evil deeds brought to bear.*

Had the investigator or counselor questioned Acer about his use of an alias name and occupation on his medical records s/he might have discovered Acer's insecurity and even paranoia about revealing his homosexuality, a sure sign of emotional conflict. Had s/he simply followed up by contacting Gutierrez who's records showed 'Johnson' had conservatively over 150 sex partners over 10 years, another indication of social and emotional instability. Had s/he followed up the issue of Acer's promiscuous sex life, as is routinely recommended by public health agency counselors who are supposed to encourage AIDS cases to notify sex partners and

*then offer support to see that all partners are informed,
educated and tested for HIV, then s/he might have
learned about Acer's preference for boys, another sure
sign of psychopathology and perversion.*

*Finally, I thought, s/he might have also learned about
Acer's alcoholism and determined his need for counseling and recovery, not continuing business as usual. Once
in recovery, mental health workers could have identified
Acer as someone who was compulsively driven to satisfy
his sexual fetishes and share his struggle with AIDS with
others.*

After mixing equal portions of water and cranberry
juice into two large glasses, I brought one to Jackie who
now sat at her desk doing paperwork. I shared my "Mon-
day morning quarterback" thoughts about Acer's missed
diagnosis.

She reminded me, "You said yourself Acer was into
power and control. He would have been motivated to
learn all about the epidemiological, medical, and legal
aspects of AIDS—to try to gain power and control over
his life threatening illness. The last thing he would have
wanted was to let the authorities take control of his dental practice."

Organizing her files, she continued, "Acer would
have also loved to exercise control over the CDC. Parsons
testified that they often spoke at length about the various
aspects of AIDS and the government's inadequate response to the epidemic. Acer had been suffering the
creeping symptoms of HIV disease for well over a year
before the Wolfrom reported he was a danger to public
health. He was well motivated to stay in practice, and he

was undoubtedly annoyed when his privacy became threatened."

I nodded in agreement still processing Jackie's arguments. A minute later I admitted, "You're right. He would have tried to avert any HRS, CDC, or dental board interference in his life and practice. According to Runnells, Acer used the fact that he was dying as a good excuse to avoid interrogation. When he did speak with investigating officials he was easily able to manipulate them with his gentle and pleasant demeanor."

I finished my drink and walked back into the kitchen to put the glass in the sink. As I did, I thought *Acer probably blinded every investigating official with his kindness and lies, just as he had done with everyone else he chose to manipulate. This could have added to his strength and resolve to conquer the greatest authorities organized health care had to offer. Once he knew they were powerless over him and that they would not heal the plague which was consuming him, he probably plotted to secure the ultimate revenge.*

The Word on the Street

As time passed, it became clearer to me that with his life threatening illness in undeniable proximity, Acer's hatred for the CDC and the American health care system probably consumed him. Parsons had told of their conversations alleging the World Health Organization (WHO) involvement in the AIDS epidemic. What he didn't mention was the fine details of these conversations which might further clarify Acer's motive for lashing out at organized medicine.

Given the potential significance of this, I decided to do some research on the "World Health Organization Theory." I figured the best place to look was in the San Francisco area in the alternative medicine arena. Over the years I had befriended several medical doctors in the Bay area who were on the cutting edge of alternative care for AIDS patients. I decided to call the director of the San Francisco Medical Research Foundation, Dr. Da Vid a physician, artist, and philosopher I had met at a National Wellness Association conference. *If anyone can tell me about the WHO theory, Da Vid could,* I reckoned.

After reconnecting with Da Vid, he consented to send me a great deal of information about the matter in question. What I learned was astonishing.

For years, the word on the street, particularly in the gay community has been that HIV is a man made virus bearing stark similarities to the Bovine Lymphotrophic Virus (BLV) cultured in cows. While the scientific community quickly moved to dispel this assertion claiming African monkeys were the source of human infection, Dr. Robert Strecker, an internist with substantial training in pathology and pharmacology insisted the virus came from bovine sources.

Research showing the similarity between HIV and the BLV finally appeared in *Nature* in 1987. Strecker, outraged that it took ten years for this work to be published, launched an all out assault on the AIDS research establishment after the majority still refused to give up the African monkey theory. According to Strecker, it was virologically absurd to believe HIV came from the monkey "since there are no genetic markers in the AIDS virus typical of the primate and the AIDS virus cannot thrive in the monkey."[6]

According to Strecker, whose work was reviewed by medical physician Jonathan Collin in a 1988 issue of *Townsend Letter for Doctors*, the AIDS virus:

Can and apparently does thrive in the cow, having essentially identical characteristics with the Bovine virus and this, further, gives a hint of the role vaccinations have played in either accidentally or purposefully inducing the AIDS epidemic.[6]

Collin reported that Strecker's research made sense, particularly considering the virology and evolution of the AIDS epidemic. Strecker's first point was that AIDS was nonexistent in Africa prior to 1975, and had it been the result of monkey bites occurring in the 1940's, as was alleged, the epidemic should have occurred in the 1960's and not late 1970's due to the twenty year timetable for case incidence doubling.[6]

More importantly, Strecker alleged the WHO launched a major African campaign against smallpox during the early 1970's which did not involve rural Pygmies, just the urban population. Had the monkey been responsible for AIDS, Strecker professed, the Pygmies of rural Africa would have had a higher incidence of AIDS than the country's urban populations. The opposite is true.

Strecker professed to have reviewed WHO research which revealed in the early 1970's their organization's scientists had studied viruses which were capable of altering the immunologic response capacity of T-lymphocytes. Strecker noted that such viruses were found in 1970, but only in some animals including sheep and cows, and that the later species is used to produce the smallpox vaccine.

Collin wrote:

Strecker remarks that it would be relatively easy to
implant such viruses in the cow carcasses used to
produce the smallpox vaccine. When the smallpox
vaccine sera was recovered from the animal carcasses, animal lymphotrophic viruses could be
carried or mutated or incorporated in the vaccine...
the epidemiology of multiple "contaminated"
smallpox vaccines given in the early 1970's would
provide exactly the right timetable for such a wide-
spread AIDS epidemic in Africa today.[6]

More pertinent to the Acer case, Strecker vigorously
promoted his theory that the AIDS virus was transmitted
to the American homosexual community during the
course of an experimental vaccination program sponsored by the United States Public Health Service in 1978.

At that time, Collin wrote:

The P.H.S. notes the recipients were sexually active,
having more than one sexual partner, and at particular risk for developing hepatitis. The homosexual populations given the vaccination were in
six major cities, including New York, San Francisco, Los Angeles, St. Louis, Houston and Chicago.
Epidemiologically, these cities now have the highest incidence of AIDS and ARC, as well as the highest death rates from AIDS.

Again, Strecker suggests that such vaccines could
easily have been contaminated with the human/
animal lymphotrophic virus and such contamina-
tion from his viewpoint was not accidental.
Strecker is convinced that this experimentation was
purposeful and that the incorporation of the
lymphotrophic virus was deployed purposely...
Strecker surmises that this is not the first time human viral experiments have led to biological disas-
ters.[6]

After reading this, I realized, *This is what Parsons meant about Acer's intense anger towards them, the government, and mainstream America. Believing in Strecker's theory, Acer undoubtedly would have blamed the U.S. Public Health Service for his disease and for infecting the entire homosexual community. He would make them pay for their treason against him and all others with AIDS.*

Suddenly it became very clear to me that *the CDC didn't find any criminal evidence implicating Acer, because they just didn't want to. If they had, the prosecution would have revealed Acer's principal motive— revenge—alerting every American and people around the world to the possibility the U.S. Public Health Service spread HIV throughout America. How incredible! He engineered a trap for the CDC—a real Catch 22—they would be damned if they investigated and discovered he was a murderer, and damned if they didn't. If they did, the world would want to know the motive. If they didn't, Acer's deeds would hold America hostage to irrational fear of AIDS and health care.*

When I shared this new found knowledge with Jackie, She paused and then shook her head in disbelief, "Wait a minute, I don't get it. You mean the CDC didn't investigate Acer as a murder suspect because they were covering up for the World Health Organization?"

"No. It's more likely they were covering up for themselves and the U.S. Public Health Service. Had they desired to solve the mystery they would have had to admit it was murder. If they admitted it was murder, everyone would have wanted to know the motive. If the motive ever got out—the fact that Acer was angry at the U.S. Public Health Service for their hepatitis B vaccine ex-

periments which allegedly brought AIDS to gay
America—then the public would freak out about vaccination programs as well as the PHS which the CDC directs."

"Do you think Acer foresaw this concern?"

"I don't see why not. He planned the whole thing
didn't he. Every bit of the little evidence found so far he
left behind on purpose. Parsons was the only gay friend
he had; he probably knew Parsons would reveal his political anger and vengeance. And so what? He would
soon be dead. He had to have realized that in order for
the CDC to expose him as a killer, they would need to
reveal to the world his principal motive. He knew they
would never do that. He had them trapped like the rats
he perceived them to be."

"I get it, his plan would assure that they would either
be disgraced in the eyes of the world, or exposed for the
crimes he believed they committed against man and society."

"Unreal! the guy was a criminal genius."

Additional Clues

Jackie and I probed further into Acer's letter and
found at least two additional clues that further revealed
his evil actions and malevolent motives.

"Here, listen to this," I announced. "At the beginning
of the fourth paragraph, he writes,"

It is with great sorrow and some surprise that I read
that I am accused of transmitting the HIV virus
(AIDS) to one of my patients.

"Note the Freudian slips?"

"Come again?"

"Pretend you were Acer for a minute. Let's say you had practiced dentistry for over a decade, and you truly 'cared for people' all your life. To 'infect anyone with this disease would be contrary to everything' you have stood for. Gradually you find yourself very ill and close to death. The next thing you know, you wake up one morning and the world is suddenly claiming a young woman was accidentally infected with your strain of HIV. Would you have written 'It is with...some surprise...' or would you be shocked as all hell?"

"I see your point. That lacks a fair amount of certainty doesn't it?"

"Why would Acer lack certainty unless he did something to make him feel uncertain? The other slip is his choice of the word 'accused'. No one was accusing him of anything at that time. No one knew how the transmission occurred—only that Bergalis and he shared the same virus!"

"You're right on. Very interesting," she admitted.

We read on and found one other clue that spoke loudly and clearly to Acer's secondary motives—his sociopathic intent to seek revenge on homophobic America, to involve mainstream Americans in his fight against AIDS, and to send shock waves of fear and confusion throughout the health care system.

"HRS investigator, Howell, did not ask Acer to use the letter as a pulpit from which to preach a correct political position or to instruct people about the psychology of AIDS, fear, and avoidance," Jackie deduced as she pointed to the part of the letter to which she was referring. "That's why it's odd that the letter states,"

> You understandably are frightened...A fear of the unknown is hard to deal with, but knowledge of what you fear can at least help you know what action to take, *if any.*

"Interesting that these statements would parallel what happened as a result of America finding out about the infections," I said, as I got up to consider the implications. "What he created was a mystery of colossal proportions which sent chills of apprehension up and down the spines of millions of people throughout America; a fear epidemic more costly and destructive than any we have ever known. He knew beforehand that people would be incapable of taking any action to reverse or resolve the harm that he had done, and they would have to live with the intense fear of the unknown generated by his unsolvable mystery."

Finally, we agreed that Acer's last deceitful claim in his open letter appeared in the last paragraph. He stated that "to infect anyone with this disease would be contrary to what I have stood for."

By this time it had become clear to us that Acer "stood for" sabotaging the CDC, the HRS, the U.S. Public Health Service, homophobes, and the American mainstream with a sociopathic agenda without regard to anyone's needs but his own. The patients he purposely selected then infected to spread AIDS and fear served him merely as human sacrifices.

The Risk of Liability and Embarrassment

Another very likely reason why the CDC blundered in the Acer investigation was because of their potential liability. Though it's very difficult to sue the U.S. government, it is possible to file a negligence suit against the HRS.

To support this theory we first evaluated the legal complaint brought against Cigna, by the Bergalises and attorney Montgomery, as recorded in detail in *AIDS in the Dental Office?*

"It's possible," I suggested to Jackie the next morning interrupting my exercise routine for a legal theory discussion, "the HRS could have pursued shutting Acer's practice down in an effort to protect the public's health, their commissioned purpose, had they suspected and documented any wrong doing." I grabbed Runnells's book off the end-table in our den and followed my wife and daughter into the kitchen.

"Maybe," said Jackie while trying to slip Alena's legs into her high chair, "but they probably didn't suspect anything."

"Someone had to suspect something after Wolfrom's report!" I urged her to consider, "Montgomery based some of his case on the fact that... here let me read it to you:"

> "Cigna Dental Health undertook to investigate Dr. Acer's office to determine a safe, sanitary and appropriate operation. Sterilization techniques were questioned..."[7]

"The HRS, CDC and/or the state dental board," I argued, "did—or at least should have undertook—to inves-

tigate Acer following the warning issued by Wolfrom to
stop him from practicing for the same reasons. In essence, Jack, official investigators should have, and failed
to, evaluate Acer's physical, mental, and emotional
health status over two months before he injected Bergalis
and the others."

"Furthermore," I continued as Alena pelted the floor
with her breakfast, "since the CDC/HRS investigator(s)
probably referred Acer for counseling regarding his use
of universal precautions, it not only have been grounds
for a law suit, at minimum it would have been tremendously embarrassing for these institutions to have made
this information known to the public."[8]

"So what you're saying is that the CDC conspired
with the HRS to:

one—keep critical information about the Acer case
investigation classified so as to avert public recognition
of Strecker's theories; two—avert a civil suit by Acer's
victims against the HRS for their oversights; and/or
three—ward off a criminal investigation which might
have publicly and politically embarrassed both CDC and
HRS investigators and officials."

"Or four—maintain the case as a mystery—most
likely an accident—in an effort to avert all the above," I
added.

"This would explain all the inconsistencies of the
cover-up," Jackie reasoned."

"Right," I said, "Give me a few minutes." I walked
over to my Mac, brought up a new document in
WordPerfect, and typed—"Inconsistencies/Cover-Up at
the HRS and CDC:

- spent more than three months investigating and blaming the victim, Kimberly Bergalis, rather than immediately investigating Acer[9];

- deleted from their official reports the negative personality profile supplied by Parsons that Acer was **very angry** and highly rebellious against the CDC, the U.S. Public Health Service, and mainstream America for their response to gays and AIDS[4];

- from the beginning, according to Jaffe, had to assume there was some kind of an accident that exposed the patient to the dentist's blood—despite the fact no other cases of doctor to patient HIV transmission had been documented[10];

- reported that Acer had been cooperative despite contradicting reports by various investigators including Jaffe[11,12] and Runnells[13];

- failed to send a dentist along with other investigators to interview Acer[1], despite the fact that their public health dentist, Dr. Robert Dumbaugh, was available and only a short distance away from Acer's office;

- speculated so imaginatively about the "accidental exposures"[4];

- failed to launch a criminal investigation of the case despite having substantial testimony that Acer was depressed, sexually aggressive and perverted; and

- why the CDC within eight months of Acer's death published guidelines for the development and use of expert panels[14] by HIV-positive health care workers to avert similar precarious situations as well as reduce such risks to the public's health in the future.[15]"

Passing the Buck

One afternoon towards the end of August, 1993 the three of us walked down to the Post Office. I had gone to the counter to purchase stamps while Jackie emptied our box. As we left the building, she handed me my issue of the *American Dental Association News* and pointed to the front page headline "Dead Suspect Means No Acer Query."[16] The article stated that no investigation was being planned since besides the lack of criminal evidence, the suspect, Acer, was dead. *ADA News* editor Julie Jacob was informed by the Martin County Sheriff's office that the State Attorney General's office felt that the case was out of its jurisdiction, and referred the case to state attorney Bruce Colton, who has jurisdiction in Stuart, Florida.

The report said, "The Florida state attorney's office cannot conduct a criminal investigation of the Dr. David Acer case because there is no one to prosecute."

"The only suspect, Dr. Acer is dead," said attorney Colton.

The articles also quoted Stephen Kindland, the spokesperson for the Florida HRS, as saying, "To try to put public misgivings to rest, we felt we needed to pursue [the criminal investigation avenue]."

However, state attorney Colton denied the formal pursuit of evidence stressing that the HRS authorities never formally requested a criminal investigation of Acer's case. "State health officials simply asked whether a criminal investigation was possible," Jacob's article went on to report.

"The medical examiners felt there were people who might know more than what they were saying," said Mr. Colton. "They felt if these people were called in under a subpoena to testify, they might open up more."

Colton also stated that if asked, his office would go over the evidence with state and federal medical investigators. "The investigation remains open," said Mr. Kindland. "If we uncover any new information, we will pursue it. For all we know, someone could step forward with new information tomorrow."

After reading the above comments several times, I offered the following analysis, "It seems to me that the Florida state attorney general's office and the HRS are attempting to hoodwink the public further and/or position themselves to pass the blame to one another in the event someone comes forward to reveal the truth. Colton's and Kindland's statements not only contradict each other, they are self incriminating.

"How?"

"Why would Colton say the case was closed 'because there was no one to prosecute,' after hearing medical investigators report their desire to 'put public misgivings to rest' and their belief that criminal evidence might be found if subpoenas were issued? Why also did Colton say the attorney general's office failed to launch a criminal inquiry because HRS investigators never formally requested the investigation? Remember what the GAO report said?"

"No, what?"

"I'll show you when we get home."

As soon as we were back at the house, I pulled out my copy of the GAO's report and read out loud:

> Because the personnel at CDC and HRS are health investigators, not criminal investigators, they brought this matter to the attention of the attorney general in Florida, but that office declined to become formally involved, noting the absence of supporting evidence.[1]

"Note they declined to get involved because of the 'absence of supporting evidence,' not the lack of a formal request or a suspect." The GAO also reported that 'both offices determined that no additional action was warranted' when Parson's incriminating testimony was forwarded to HRS and through them to the Florida attorney general's office."

"I still don't get it."

"Given the fact that the personnel at the HRS are 'not criminal investigators,' why would the attorney general have authorized HRS investigators to interview Ed Parsons when they knew it concerned Acer's alleged criminal activity?"

"Oh yeah, good question."

"Why also was the testimony about Acer's drunken, sloppy, and aggressive behavior given by another gay acquaintance not reported by any government investigators, only by Runnells?"[17]

"Another good question."

"Why also would Kindland say, 'If we uncover any new information, we will pursue it,' when they ignored the descriptive data and existence of Acer's gay acquaintances."

"I don't know."

Why also would Kindland report that 'the investigation remains open' when Colton says it's closed?"

"Tell me already!"

"So long as the investigation remains open to the HRS they can continue to claim they're doing their best, and continue to withhold self-incriminating evidence which might be made available through the Freedom of Information Act if they were to close the case. The attorney general's office, on the other hand, by pronouncing the case closed can assure that no additional evidence will be sought or found."

"And if someone does come forward with the truth, the two of them could use each other as scapegoats."

"Right!"

Other Possible Excuses and Reasons for the Mystery

At this point in our investigation, Jackie and I were still open to consider any other reason the CDC and HRS might not have wanted to solve the case. We packed up Alena, rations, and beach toys, and drove to Good Harbor Beach for a few hours of rest, relaxation and contemplation. Within a few minutes we were building sand castles and once again considering the case.

"Giving CDC and HRS investigators all the benefit of doubt, it might have been an honest oversight that they concluded the deadly exposures were all accidents," Jackie proposed. "Don't you think the CDC and HRS investigators could have been blinded by Acer's deception, and simply became confused when they attempted to research this case?"

"You're being extremely kind. I think they're a lot smarter than that. Scientists would have been more thoughtful in both questioning Acer, Parsons and others, and in analyzing the results of their probe. I'm appalled they would delete vital data from their research reports, and at minimum I believe they should be cited for scientific misconduct."

"You know what their excuse will be?"

"What?"

"That they didn't have the expertise to do anything but a public health investigation."

"You're probably right. But, that should have been more reason to involve the Florida attorney general's office from the beginning of the investigation."

Alena was now destroying our castle as quickly as Jackie and I could repair it. I then recalled Jaffe's comments to the press.

"You know, in July '91 Jaffe reported that a criminal investigation would probably follow their frustrated efforts.[15] But, as mentioned in the GAO report, Butterworth, or some other state attorney, nixed the idea allegedly due to a lack of criminal evidence.[1] What I don't get is faced with an unsolved mystery affecting the entire American health care system and public health in general, why would Butterworth and the CDC wait for criminal evidence to suddenly, years later, appear, when the purpose of criminal investigations is to uncover this type of evidence immediately?"

"Me neither."

I continued dribbling wet sand to make a turret, "It just doesn't make sense unless you consider an organized cover-up." A minute later another reason dawned on me. "It's also possible that the CDC saw this case as a fabulous opportunity to use the news media along with public and professional apprehension about the mystery to help to promote one of their top priority causes—persuading health care and public safety personnel to comply with universal precautions."

"That's possible," Jackie admitted. "If everyone knew Acer deliberately infected his patients, then many dentists and physicians would argue, "Nothing ever happened before, so why should I adopt all these difficult and costly infection control practices?""

"You got it. But it's interesting to note, that the CDC keeps using the threat of death and dying, unsuccessfully I might add, to get the people— including health professionals—to change risky habits. Think about it; their two essential messages are both fear based. One is essentially, 'You use IV drugs—you will die,' and the other is 'You have unprotected sex—you will die.'

"For health professionals that translates into, 'You practice without taking universal precautions—both you and your patients may die.'"

"Exactly. So you see, the CDC couldn't have paid for a better fear campaign to sensitize health and safety personnel and the general public at the same time to the need for improved infection control behaviors. Unfortunately, the runaway media caused everyone to become overly, irrationally, and neurotically anxious about the risk of receiving health care and treating HIV-positive patients."

We spent the rest of the afternoon taking turns chasing Alena about the beach, body surfing, and sun worshipping. As the day passed I kept trying to think of another reason why the HRS and CDC may not have wanted the case resolved. Intuitively I knew something else remained to be discovered.

Chapter 11.
Where's The Beef?
Finding The Hard Evidence

On the drive back home from Gloucester, a feeling of frustration came over me. I turned to Jackie and said, "You know, so far we haven't learned anything that might hold up in a court of law. You can't nail 'murder one' on a suspect without having hard evidence with which to go to court, can you?"

"So where does the prosecution currently stand?"

Well, first we learned that from the beginning of the "deadly innocence" case, the CDC wrongly assumed it had been an accident, and that their official investigation reports were principally bogus, replete with ludicrous assumptions and mistaken theories about the ways the exposures might have happened. Essentially, we learned that the only plausible explanation of how HIV transmission from Dr. Acer to at least six of his patients could have taken place was by intent. We learned that public health service officials, CDC directors, and Florida HRS investigators neglected, deleted, overlooked, and/or intentionally covered up, in their official reports, vital facts intimating murder. We learned that several factors including threatened public health, money, politics, threatened public image, and/or gross ineptitude probably caused the CDC investigators to fail to disclose the hidden facts about the case and solve the mystery. We also learned that this official misdirection not only cost American taxpayers dearly but also cost the health and

lives of tens of thousands of people who became innocent victims of the media driven "fear-of-AIDS-epi-
demic."

"O.K., now what about Acer?"

"Acer was a highly unstable person. We learned that
he had several potential motives for selecting and then
infecting at least six mainstream American patients.
Among his motivations was his vendetta against the CDC
and the U.S. Public health care system for allegedly infecting gays with HIV contaminated hepatitis vaccines
and for not creating a cure for AIDS soon enough to save
him from being disgraced in the eyes of his mother, and
from dying. We also learned that Acer maintained extreme hostility towards American society for being generally homophobic since this made him and other
homosexuals feel insecure and persecuted for being gay.
We learned that he probably suffered tremendous guilt
that he had remained a closet homosexual who felt too
embarrassed and insecure to participate in gay rights
demonstrations and equal rights politics—and that in his
mind, giving lethal injections to selected patients might
reserve for him a place in health care, AIDS awareness,
and gay rights history."

"SO WHAT AGAIN! You need more than
psychobabble and a few good motives to resolve the
case."

"Your right. I need to produce something really solid
to link the suspect to the crime, or I need something in
writing which shows the CDC or HRS actually did what
seems obvious to us."

"It will be impossible to produce a murder weapon,
since Acer easily discarded the essential pieces of evi-

dence and there were no witnesses."

"You're right, the case doesn't look good. Maybe that's what I'm feeling. The American public may remain irrationally anxious about health care in the age of AIDS unless they believe beyond a reasonable doubt that Acer was responsible for these deadly deeds."

"So what's our next move?"

"I don't know."

Tracking a Criminal Psychologist

Since Acer was dead and I lacked substantive evidence with which to prove my case, my next step was to show that Acer's personality profile (see Table 1) equaled someone who was prone to commit murder—or infect others with HIV. Then I might be a lot closer to providing evidence beyond a reasonable doubt that Acer intentionally infected his patients.

My next step was to conduct research into the psychology of criminals, specifically serial killers. Having never studied criminal psychology nor known anyone who had, I began by placing telephone calls to local law enforcement organizations.

The first call I made was to the Massachusetts State Police Academy. After several unsuccessful attempts to connect with anyone there knowledgeable about criminal psychology, I was referred to the Director of Training's office. Unfortunately, he never returned my call.

The next day, I pulled out my 1990 edition of *The Directory of Experts Authorities, and Spokespersons* to see if anyone listed might be able to help me gain access to some criminal psychology literature. Here I found under the listing "Psychology of Law" the name Jim Kolesar, Director of Public Information from Williams College in Williamstown, MA. Mr. Kolesar returned my call within an hour.

I asked him, "Do you have anyone there I might be able to speak with regarding criminal psychology?" He said that he didn't, however, he suggested that I give the FBI Academy in Quantico, Virginia a call. He said that they had a behavioral science unit and that most likely they would have what I was looking for.

After getting the telephone number for the FBI, I was about to dial when it struck me. *What if they're in on the 'cover-up,'* I thought. Though I didn't think this was a likely possibility, having grown up in Southern New Jersey with my father, a politician, I knew that stranger things have been known to happen. I therefore decided not to tell the FBI why I needed the information.

Upon calling the Behavioral Science Unit of the FBI Academy, and explaining who I was and what I was looking for, I was immediately impressed by the warmth and genuine interest expressed by the individual on the other end of the line. Our conversation went something like this:

"I'm looking for any scientific research you can send me on criminal psychology particularly related to the psychology of serial killers or mass murderers," I said.

"What do you do?" the person asked.

"I'm a dentist," I automatically blurted without thinking and immediately I regretted it. *Not good! That may clue them into my investigation of the Acer case*, I thought.

"This is a pretty odd request for a dentist, isn't it?" she queried.

I knew I had to think of something really fast so I said, "Well, I'm a pretty odd dentist. I have a master's degree in public health from Harvard University, and I'm involved in a behavioral science research project."

She immediately dropped the interrogation and became cordial and interested in helping once again. *Phew!* I thought, *That was close.*

She then informed me that they had a number of publications which might be related to the topic I was studying and that the materials would be mailed out the same afternoon.

"Thank you very much," I said, "I really appreciate your help."

Two days later, Jackie had taken Alena to Boston and left me alone. A child modelling agency, and a toy manufacturer had requested her for a screening. That morning our mail lady Debbie arrived with a gray-brown envelope from the FBI bearing an assortment of documents including a list of "Publications of the National Center for the Analysis of Violent Crimes," and a 141 page bulletin titled, *Criminal Investigative Analysis: Sexual Homicide.* My first glance at this title was followed by the thought, *What did they send me this for? I didn't ask for anything related to sexual homicide.* So I opened this book first.

As though guided by a higher power, my thumb opened to page 39, and in front of my eyes was the title, "Sexual Homicide: A Motivational Model" by Ann W. Burgess, Carol R. Hartman, Robert K. Ressler, John E. Douglas, and Arlene McCormack.[1] The words "motivation model" in the title struck me at once as fascinating since these were the two words I had used to title several of my previous publications describing my "Self-Care Motivation Model" for healthy human development. I immediately read the abstract:

> The findings from this exploratory study are reported in terms of the descriptive background characteristics of 36 sexual murderers, their behavior and experiences in connection with their developmental stages, and the central role of sadistic fantasy and critical cognitive structures that support the act of sexual murder. A five-phase motivational model is presented.[1]

Wow! How interesting, I thought. *This would be a good article for me to read to get oriented to the field of criminal psychology, particularly since I can totally relate to the application of motivational models to explain behaviors and experiences associated with developmental stages in life. Also, since this article includes research on the "descriptive background characteristics of 36 sexual murderers this might show me how to analyze the descriptive data I now have on Acer. Maybe some of the factors associated with being a sexual murderer will match some of the Acer data as well.* I had absolutely no idea just how this would change the course of our investigation.

Chapter 12.
The FBI Sexual
Homicide Report

I immediately began reading the report by Ann Burgess and her team[1], highlighting in yellow the sections which represented new lessons for me or information which seemed related to the analysis of data I had on Acer.

For decades the report said, motiveless murders have baffled law enforcers and mental health professionals.[2] Serial killers often did their dirty work leaving little if any evidence behind and virtually no clues to define a motive for their slayings. Although serial killers have existed throughout history, the researchers reported, the prevalence of mortality by unjustifiable homicide has never been greater.[1,3]

The group explained why law enforcement professionals often turn to behavioral science experts when they are unable to determine intent in a murder case. Burgess and her co-workers reported that:

> FBI agents have found that they need to understand the thought patterns of murderers in order to make sense of crime scene evidence and victim information. Characteristics of evidence and victims can reveal much about the murderer's intensity of planning, preparation, and follow-through. From these observations, the agents begin to uncover the murderer's motivation, recognizing how dependent

motivation is to the killer's dominant thinking patterns. In many instances, a hidden, sexual motive emerges, a motive that has its origins in fantasy.[1]

In essence, sexual killers they explained, represent a unique class of violent criminals who kill for the sake of power, control, aggressive brutality, and sexuality. The murderers in such cases are commonly diagnosed as sexual sadists who gain pleasure from both sexual practices that are socially prohibited as well as from inflicting pain and suffering on their victims.[2] They use their highly active imaginations to plan, carry out, and recall their criminal actions, and they repeatedly rejoice in the gruesome details of their recollections.[3]

Given this knowledge, the Burgess group sought to develop their "Motivational Model for Sexual Homicide," which incorporated all of the psychological-social and developmental factors they discovered including the motivations, behaviors, and personality characteristics which would help sexual homicide investigators identify the murderers and their patterns of criminal activity.

One important realization that I gained immediately is that "the data set" the FBI investigators had collected, for each of thirty-six sexual killers,

> Consisted of the best available data from two types of sources: official records (psychiatric and criminal records, pretrial records, court transcripts, and prison records) and interviews with the offenders.[4]

This is essentially identical to the sources of data Runnells, the CDC, and I had collected to describe Acer's personal and behavioral history. I thought. The only difference is, they used criminal and/or prison records and we had medical records and testimonials provided by his dental office staff, patients, and others who knew him.

The one disclaimer the FBI investigators made early on in this report is that this study was not to be used to predict or generalize childhood or adolescent experiences, but was specifically designed to help in the analysis of subsequent "sexual and 'motiveless' murders." I read on intently.

The next section of the report described their findings. They stated that the thirty-six sexual killers in their study,

> Began their lives with certain advantages. Most of them grew up in the 1940s and 1950s, a period when attitudes in the United States favored oldest, white male children; all subjects were male, the majority (thirty-three) were white, and many were eldest sons.[5]

Acer was born on November 11, 1949, and was the oldest white male son of four children in all—two from a former and two from a latter marriage, I recalled.

The FBI investigators reported that the killers,

> Were of good intelligence, with 29% classified in the average range, 36% in the bright normal and superior range, and 15% in the very superior range. These attributes fostered in the offenders a certain sense of privilege and entitlement.[5]

I remembered, *Acer had maintained a B average throughout college and dental school. He was intelligent and scientifically trained.* The way Acer had responded with consistent denial regarding his HIV status and progressive illness plus his statement to his father that he had hoped to be cured by the CDC's discovery of a vaccine before having to break the news to his parents,[6,7] made me stop and question, *Was this the same sense of entitlement that the killers had?*

"Initially," the FBI investigators continued,

The majority of men began life in two-parent homes. Half of the mothers were homemakers; three-quarters of the fathers earned stable salaries. Over 80% of the offenders described their family socioeconomic levels as average (self-sufficient) or better. Thus mothers were in the home raising the children; fathers were earning stable incomes; poverty was not a factor in the financial status of families.[5]

This is consistent with Acer's early childhood, I thought.

" Although the families initially appeared to be functional with both parents present," the FBI report stated, "problems were noted within the parents' backgrounds. Families had criminal (50.0%), psychiatric (53.3%), alcohol abuse (69.0%), drug abuse (33.3%), or sexual (46.2%) problems in their histories."[5]

Though Acer may have been born into a relatively functional family, I considered, *the fact that he abused alcohol suggests that he was possibly a child of at least one alcoholic. It seems to me that his family would have had sexual problems in dealing with David's latent homosexuality.* I continued reading.

It appears that parents of these men were often absorbed in their own problems. Thus, while being offered little guidance because of their parents' preoccupation with their troubles, the murderers as young boys were witness to these deviant role patterns of criminal behavior, substance abuse, and poor interpersonal relationships.[8]

I recalled that Acer, became the early victim of a broken home when his father died. His mother, undoubtedly needing to cope with the stress of raising two young boys without a husband, probably needed to turn her attention away from David for three reasons: 1) David's younger brother Bruce required the bulk of her attention,

2) Mrs. Acer was not financially independent, and she needed to think about her economic well being, and 3) She desired to remarry, thus she would have had to spend a fair amount of time dating or courting in one (or more) new relationship(s).

"In 47% of cases," the FBI report continued,

The father left the home before the subject was 12; in 43% of the cases at least one parent was absent at some time prior to the subjects reaching age 18. This loss of the father required many of the offenders to adjust to a new male caretaker during childhood and adolescent years.[8]

What a coincidence, I thought. *This is exactly what happened in David Acer's early childhood.*

In addition, the report stated that,

Instability in the family residence was also noted in many cases (68%). In addition, 40% of the subjects lived outside the family home before age 18. Locations included foster homes, state homes, detention centers, and mental hospitals. The histories of frequent moving reduced the boys' opportunities to develop positive outside relationships that might have compensated for family instability.[8]

Though the Acer family has refused to be interviewed on the subject of David's early life beyond what Runnells was able to gather, I realized the possibility that *Harriett Acer may have had David stay with someone else following her husband's death or sometime thereafter to reduce some of her stress. Runnells did mention that David did move from three homes before he left for college.*

Examination of performance behaviors of the subjects revealed that despite their intelligence and potential in many areas, performance in academics, employment, and military was often poor."[8]

Though this was apparently not the case for David Acer, the FBI investigators went on to say that, "one-third did average or better in school."

David could have easily fallen into this third of the group, I considered.

The final demographic and historical antecedent found among the group of thirty-six sexual killers was evidence of child abuse. The FBI researchers noted in the histories of the study sample, thirteen of thirty-one killers were physically abused, twenty-three of thirty-one were psychologically abused, and twelve of twenty-eight had been sexually abused as children.

In addition, the FBI investigators determined, the top eleven most common behaviors of the sexual killers during adulthood in descending order of frequency were: 1) assaultive to adults (86%), daydreaming (81%), masturbation (81%), isolation (73%), rebelliousness (72%), chronic lying (68%), poor body image (62%), stealing (56%), nightmares (52%), sleep problems (50%), and phobias (24%).

The internal behaviors most consistently reported (from childhood through adulthood) are daydreaming, compulsive masturbation, and isolation. The external behaviors most consistently reported include chronic lying, rebelliousness, stealing, cruelty to children, and assault on adults.[9]

That's remarkable, I thought, as I immediately noted a remarkable similarity between Dr. Acer's frequently reported behaviors and those of the sexual killers the FBI group had studied.

It was as if the glove of data I had on Acer fit nearly perfectly with a very bizarre and unique group of individuals the FBI had identified as sexual killers. *But that doesn't make sense*, I thought, *Acer didn't have sex with his patients before he injected them. What's the deal?*

I read through the next section of the FBI report which discussed the role of fantasy in these criminals' lives, how in order to escape a difficult and traumatic childhood, most of them withdrew from society, became isolated loners, and in their quiet isolation fantasized vividly and profusely about an alternate reality in which they were all powerful, knowing, and in control of events.

This section of the report fascinated me since I was very familiar with the powerful role that imagery plays in determining behaviors and life outcomes. In fact, I had published several scientific reports on the use of guided imagery and relaxation to help anxious dental patients overcome their irrational fears, and had personally befriended two of the pioneers in the field of using imagery as a tool for healing and behavior change: Dr. Thomas Stampfl from the University of Wisconsin, and a neighbor of mine, Dr. Joe Cautela, of Gloucester, MA.

This section struck me like a lightening bolt. *This is David Acer exactly! He spent his life in a fantasy world rather than in the real world.*

One indelible observation that Runnells recorded was that Acer couldn't even socialize when he wanted to:

Although he was a member of his dental society, he seldom attended meetings. Mostly, he was remembered as attending Christmas parties, where he 'just stood around-alone.'[10]

Can you imagine going to Christmas parties and always standing around alone? *The guy had to be fantasizing,* I thought. *He was probably having a great time in his head!*

It also occurred to me what a great occupation dentistry is for someone who enjoys fantasizing. As a clinical dentist in practice for over sixteen years, I can tell you that providing dental care is often so routine that your mind can't help but drift happily away into some pleasant fantasy—if you're a normal dentist. For Acer, what he was imagining while practicing dentistry or socializing with "friends" was unfathomable.

The FBI investigators reported,

In analyzing the data we obtained through interviews with the murderers, we attempted to link our quantifiable findings with indications from the murderers themselves of long-standing, aggressive thoughts and fantasies directed toward sexualized death. The findings suggest that these thought patterns were established early and existed in a context of social isolation.[11]

Is this consistent with the socially isolated life that everyone observed Acer to lead—the quiet, reserved, independent, and withdrawn person everyone testified about, I wondered?

The investigators also discussed the development of negative, aggressive, and sexualized fantasy during the childhood and adulthood of sexual murderers,

As children, the murderers often thought of other children and family members as extensions of their inner worlds.

This might have been related to Acer's intensely protective and defensive relationship with his mother, I considered.

They revealed intermittent awareness of the impact of their early childhood behavior on others. They were not influenced by the response of others to their behavior.[11]

These fantasy and real life behaviors continued to be repeated throughout adolescence and adulthood the investigators stated.

Regarding sexual and aggressive fantasies impacting serial killing behavior, the FBI investigators commonly found these patterns were associated with repeatedly acting out the aggressions and sexual violence the killer had sustained or witnessed during childhood. They described one killer who:

At age 15 took younger boys into the bathroom of his residential facility and forced oral and anal sex on them, reenacting his own victimization at age 10 but reversing his role from victim to victimizer. However, he did not consciously connect this behavior with his own earlier assaults. The assaultive rituals were his attempts at mastery and control over people and situations.[12]

I could not help but think, *was this like Acer's reported compulsive desire to get drunk, find gay men and boys, aggressively come on and have sex with them? Could this have been driven by similar forces and sexual fantasies?*

I was still unconvinced, however, that Acer was a
sexual murderer. I couldn't see how the dynamics of
Acer's case and the Florida dental tragedy fit with the
image I always had in my mind about sexual killers.
Again, Acer didn't sexually abuse his dental patient victims. In fact, nothing at all appeared sexual about their
relationships so how could he have been a sexual killer?

Chapter 13.
Motivating
Sexual Homicide

The rest of the FBI report by Ann Burgess and her group discussed the workings of a brilliant "motivational model of sexual homicide." (See Figure 1.)

Based on the information they had collected, the investigators theorized that the:

> Murderers early development of an active, aggressive fantasy life (daydreams) combined with later sexual reinforcement (compulsive masturbation [or possibly climactic satisfaction gained during homosexual encounters in Acer's case]) and increasing detachment from social rules of conduct (social isolation [which everyone observed of Acer]) provide a framework that reinforces his subsequent violent behavior.[1]

They then began to describe their model as having:

> Five basic interacting components including: (1) the murderer's ineffective social environment, (2) child and adolescent formative events, (3) patterned responses to these events, (4) resultant actions towards others, and (5) the killer's reactions, via a mental 'feedback filter' to his murderous acts.[1]

I thought it was an incredible coincidence that the "self-care motivation model" I developed also had "five basic interacting components."

This is unbelievable, I thought as the recognition struck me, *Their "motivational model for sexual homi-*

tially THE POLAR OPPOSITE of my "self-care motivation model" for healthy human development! Whereas theirs describes what happens to an innocent child to make him a cold-hearted killer, mine describes what it takes for a child to become an optimally healthy, happy, productive, and loving human being. This is unreal! I sat back to appreciate the majesty of the moment.

Ineffective Social Environment

According to child development theorists, the quality of child-parent relationships and the strength or quality of a child's bonding with parents ultimately determines how the child later learns to interact with others throughout life. In essence, quality social relationships and loving interactions in adult life depend on whether, as a child, the person was able to experience full bonding and a high quality relationship with his parents. As the FBI researchers explained,

> One of the primary functions of family life is to develop a child who has a positive bonding with his social environment.[1]

In their populations of murderers however, this social bonding failed or became confined and selective. The killers parents or caretakers either ignored, rationalized, or normalized their children's behaviors while they were growing up because of their own problems such as substance abuse--alcoholism, for example. This supported their developing distortions and perceptions about reality. The parents or caretakers of the killers failed to provide nurturing and protection. Instead, they imposed adult expectations on the boys such as, "Boys should be strong and take care of themselves." The killers, as children, may have been reprimanded and even brought to court, but they tended to normalize the action as in,

> 'All boys get into trouble.' The ineffective social environment expands from caretakers to individuals in a community whose work brings them into contact with the young person (e.g., teachers, counselors, ministers, police).[2]

Given his psychological, social and sexual confusion along with parents who found it most difficult to accept homosexuality—essentially who he was, Acer likewise had at least a partially ineffective family life as a young child. With the death of his father and birth of his younger brother, perhaps his mother could not give him the care he needed. Again, given his homosexuality, it would have been difficult for him to bond with his stepfather or any male father figure. Perhaps this was symbolized by Acer continuing to hold on to his dead father's name, "Johnson." *How ironic,* I thought, *he would use this only when trying to hide his true identity.*

Also, the fact that Acer's mother's defensive insistence that David had been completely independent, despite the fact that he depended on her advice so often, may have reflected his struggle for family connection despite his compulsion towards social isolation.

I recalled Harriett Acer's insistence that David "was not a mama's boy" and questioned, *Might this suggest the imposition of adult expectations as was commonly found among sexual killers? Had Harriet and Victor Acer been homophobic, as Runnells suggested, the young, gay David would have probably been reprimanded for any effeminate actions. He would have felt pressured by parental and social attitudes that homosexuality was "a sin against God," and felt guilty about his homosexuality. Might he have tried to normalize his behaviors in order to please his family and survive in a largely homophobic society?* I questioned.

Formative Events

FBI researchers identified three key factors that contributed to the early development of sexual killers. The experience of trauma in the form of physical or sexual abuse was the first. As children, they reported, sexual killers commonly encounter normal traumas such as illness and death, non-normal traumas including physical and/or sexual abuse, and/or indirect trauma including witnessed family violence.

> Within the context of the child's ineffective social environment, the child's distress caused by the trauma is neglected. The child is neither protected nor assisted in recovery from the abusive and overwhelming events.[2]

I recalled that Acer's relationship with his mother was quite unique and suggested the existence of mutual defensiveness and protectiveness. Again the questions came to mind. *Were both mother and son physically and/ or sexually assaulted? Did they need to rely on one another to guard themselves against an offender? If this occurred, and Harriett Acer had practiced denial as a coping mechanism, then David would have been ineffectively helped to express his feelings and concerns. Therefore, he would have been expected to become socially withdrawn and to develop a pattern of habitually repressing his feelings and emotions.*

I continued to question, *Had such a trauma occurred, would Harriett Acer have expected David to be able to handle such a trauma independently and not like a "mama's boy?" Could she have said something like, "Hush! We won't talk about it—just let it go?" Might this have unintentionally encouraged David to develop distorted perceptions about normal social interactions as well as provide the lack of nurturing that is indicative of aggressive, antisocial, sexually deviant, and ultimately homicidal adult behavior?*

In addition, the report went on to say that:

The child's memories of frightening and upsetting life experiences shape the child's developing thought patterns. The type of thinking that emerges develops structured, patterned behaviors that in turn help generate daydreams and fantasies... Successful resolution of traumatic events results in the child being able to talk about the event in the past tense and with equanimity. Unsuccessful resolution of the trauma underscores the victim's helplessness and often with the emergence of aggressive fantasies aimed at achieving the dominance and control absent from reality.[2,3,4]

The second factor associated with the formative events part of the FBI's sexual homicide model is the failure of the child to develop normally due to the lack of bonding to his caregivers. In many cases, they stated,

Where the child has been psychologically deprived or neglected, he may feel a diminished emotional response.[5]

That's just what was reported by Acer's patients, I thought.

Sherry Johnson had commented to reporters that Acer showed no remorse and expressed no apology after inflicting her with pain.[6]

Months later, Barbara Webb told Maury Povich, on national television, when asked if Acer conversed much, "Oh, no. He was the most boring man I've ever met in my life."

During the same show Povich questioned Lisa Shoemaker, another Acer victim, "Never asked about you, never conversed, never socialized?"

"No, and I was terrified... I tried to crack jokes to try to break the ice for myself, and he didn't even react... He just existed. He came in and worked on my teeth and left."

Not long after Povich's show, during a *20/20* segment aired on October 1, 1993, Barbara Walters asked Parsons if he ever questioned Acer about intentionally infecting his patients. Parsons said yes. "He didn't respond which is why I, at that time, felt that there was something wrong. It just seemed to me that what I was looking for was some concern, and it struck me extremely strange at that point."[7]

"Are you sure now that Dr. Acer did this deliberately? You have no concrete proof?" Walters asked.

"I have a personal experience with the man, and conversations, and I really believe that that's sufficient for me. He never denied he infected them and I would assume that if an individual accidentally infected someone with a life threatening virus that there would be some concern or some remorse. And the complete lack of that concerned me then and it concerns me of course today," Parsons replied.[7]

Interpersonal failure is the third factor in this part of the FBI model. This is the:

Failure of the caretaking adult to serve as a role model for the developing child. There are various reasons for this failure including the caretaker being absent or serving as an inadequate role model.[5]

Such failures include one or more caretakers who are either abusive or use drugs including alcohol. It was common for the sexual killer to have experienced violence in the home such as drunken fights and/or aggression associated with sexual events.

We may never know if this occurred in the Acer family, I thought.

Patterned Responses

The third part of the FBI "motivational model for sexual homicide," the development of patterned responses, includes:

Two subcategories: (1) critical personal traits, and (2) cognitive mapping and processing [that is, thought patterns and processes]. These subcategories interact with each other to generate fantasies.[5]

During normal child development, positive personality characteristics such as warmth, honesty, trust, and security help a child to connect with others. These critical traits along with effective family or social support, help the child develop proficiency and autonomy.

In the group of sexual killers, however, the FBI investigators found,

There was a propensity for the 36 men to develop negative rather than positive personality traits. These negative personal traits interfere with the formation of social relationships and the development of an emotional capacity within the context of human encounters. Increased social isolation encourages a reliance on fantasy as a substitute for human encounter. In turn, individual personality development becomes dependent on the fantasy life and its dominant themes, rather than on social interaction. With human encounters and negotiations, there is failure to develop the corresponding social values, such as respect for others' lives and property.[5]

The critical personal traits the sexual homicide investigators found among the thirty-six men they studied included chronic lying, rebelliousness, aggression, social isolation, preferences for autoerotic activities and fetishes—that is compulsions such as intense physical and/or sexual drives—and a sense of entitlement:

> The offender's chronic lying underscores their lack of trust and commitment to a world of rules and negotiation. Rather, distrust and a sense of entitlement to whatever they can get dominate their perceptions. Their social isolation and aggression interact, restricting sexual development based on caring, pleasure, and companionship. Because they are so isolated, the men have little opportunity for interpersonal experiences that might modify their misconceptions about themselves and others. Their personal affective lives (that is, their ability to feel and/or master the emotional part of themselves) become dependent on fantasy for development. In turn, fantasy becomes the primary source of emotional arousal and that emotion is a confused mixture of sex and aggression.[5]

All at once, I had the instantaneous realization, *this is David Acer they're talking about!*

I read the paragraph again and realized, *this is the reason why Acer couldn't remain socially stable or sexually monogamous. The fact that his dental office victims were not sexually molested didn't mean anything! He felt justi-*

fied to use them for a "higher" purpose—to get at the CDC and teach them as well as mainstream America a lesson they would never forget. And his sense of entitlement allowed him to take these innocent lives without remorse. That's exactly how he was with the HRS and CDC investigators as well. "Don't bother me with your dying dental patients, and unsolvable mystery," Acer probably thought, "I'm dying and I'm entitled to die in peace."

I continued to read in amazement:

Cognitive mapping refers to the structure and development of thinking patterns that give both control and development to one's internal life (e.g., one's sense of self) and link the individual to the social environment (e.g., one's interpretation of others and beliefs about the world). The process of cognitive mapping generates the meaning of events for an individual and mediates sensory arousal patterns. Additionally, it is a filtering system that allows for interpretation of new information (e.g., "It's my life and I can live it my way.")[5]

It seemed to me that this echoed the attitude expressed by Acer when he refused to stop practicing dentistry or quit drinking. Even his disregard for proper infection control practices reflected this attitude.

Cognitive mapping and processing are aimed at self-preservation and equilibrium through the reduction of the negative affects of helplessness, terror, and pervasive anxiety.[5]

Could this be how Acer's fantasy plan for revenge against the CDC was reinforced, I reflected. He rationalized all of his frightening thoughts and behaviors in order to be able to live with himself.

All his thought patterns, mental and emotional pro-
cesses, and behaviors were oriented towards preserving
a positive self-concept. I can see that's essentially what
Runnells and Jaffe reported when they said that Acer's
story was one of deception and self-interest.

It seemed to me that Acer's drive towards self-preservation, coupled with his sense of entitlement, could have
spurred his anger, hatred, and rebelliousness. By infecting his patients and then linking the mystery to the CDC's
guidelines, as expressed in his letter, this all seemed part
of a calculated plan for revenge. It would also teach the
CDC, all of health care, and mainstream America what it
felt like to be helpless, terrorized, suffer from pervasive
anxiety, and die from AIDS. *That's exactly the outcome*
produced, I reflected.

"I don't know whether this man was just a monster or
whether he had some kind of messiah complex whereby he
was going to bring the attention of the world to the AIDS
field where the (infected) grandmothers and the young
people would make people notice this is spreading and this
is real," lamented Barbara Webb. "But why the hell he
would have to pick on people who were young; who had
their whole lives ahead of them, cause that's just not fair "[7]

"In the murderers," the FBI researchers continued,

> The mapping is repetitive and lacking socially en-
> hancing cognitions [thoughts], moving the indi-
> vidual to an antisocial position and view of the
> world. What emerges is a primary sense of entitle-
> ment to express oneself regardless of its impact on
> others. The thought and action are justified through
> the cognitive mapping of the murderer. The indi-
> vidual does not experience a positive impact with
> the social environment. This occurs because his
> fantasies and thinking patterns are a substitute for

social relationships. They are designed to stimulate and reduce tension. A sense of self is developed and bolstered by the fantasies. The self-image is terrifying to imagined others and contributes to further social isolation. The process continues and becomes the primary source of energy for the psychological life of the individual. Imagined outcomes of control and dominance over others become a substitute for a sense of mastery of internal and external experience.[5]

Now I could see how and why Acer was compelled to do what he did. His greatest desire after realizing that it was too late—the CDC was not going to find a vaccine or a cure for AIDS—would have been to pay them back for his pain, anxiety, and suffering. *This was probably the only joy left for him,* I theorized, *everything else was coming to an end. His physical body was decaying; he was no longer capable of disguising his disease to take further advantage of indiscriminate sex with men and boys. With a warped desire to gain emotional pleasure through the domination and control of his enemies, he would have infected his patients with no feeling and no remorse.*

The dynamics of cognitive mapping and processing, according to the FBI report include, nightmares, fantasies, daydreams, and thoughts with strong visual elements. The investigators explained,

There is internal dialogue [self-talk] of limiting beliefs regarding cause, effect, and probability. The subjects deal in absolutes and generalizations. The themes of their fantasies include dominance, revenge, violence, rape, molestation, power, control, torture, mutilation, inflicting pain on self/others, and death. High sensory arousal levels become the preferred state. The preoccupation with the aggressive themes, the detailed cognitive [mental] activity, and elevated kinesthetic [physical sensational] arousal states eventually move the person into action.[8]

I was fascinated by the next section of the FBI report which dealt with the biochemistry of sexual killers. The researchers evaluated the neurochemical and hormonal links to homicidal thinking and fantasizing. The scientists argued that natural mood elevating drugs manufactured by the body have been found in marathon runners, surgery patients, and more recently in people who engage in self-mutilation. They theorized that both internal as well as environmental stress could elicit the release of opium-like chemicals in killers. Experiments had shown that the removal of such stressors actually caused people to go through withdrawal—associated with malaise, anxiety, and irritability. This mental, emotional, and chemical mechanism, they reported, is also present in those who suffer from post-traumatic stress (PTS).

To avoid having to go through withdrawal as well as to maintain their pleasure state, killers, they said, replay their deadly deeds in their minds and tune into news reports about the offense. They also seek additional thrills by repeating the offense which renews their feeling of excitement, pleasure, or elation. If not, they suffer from withdrawal."[8]

In essence, serial killers are compelled to kill to gain pleasure and avoid emotional pain and depression. Whereas most people focus on doing good things for others to give and gain pleasure, sexual murderers do just the opposite.

Runnells and the government investigators argued that Acer's friends, patients, and family described him as a "very kind" and "gentle" man who stood for serving people through the practice of dentistry. "He couldn't have done it!" they argued.

But now I could see that Acer's occupation and his very kind and gentle appeal could have been a front for him to covertly gain pleasure from the pain and torment he inflicted. Runnells wrote,

> Acer was very effective in portraying the image he wanted the public to accept.[9]

Bob actually hit the nail on the head, I realized, but lacking a behavioral science background, couldn't see how meaningful his descriptive data and observations actually were.

There were several patient accounts which indicated Acer's warped sense of gaining pleasure besides Sherry Johnson's traumatic account for which Acer shared no apology and showed no remorse. Runnells provided other dreadful Acer/patient experiences in *AIDS in the Dental Office?*[10] Apparently, Acer had the reputation as being a "tooth puller." One patient recalled Acer suggested that she have her tooth pulled. After seeking a second opinion, the tooth was saved by the second dentist through simple gum treatments.

In a most bizarre account, Runnells documented one experience Barbara Webb had during the extraction of her upper front tooth. Any dentist will tell you that extractions of upper front teeth, particularly in older people, are commonly the easiest extractions you can do—particularly for dentists who have been extracting teeth in the military and general practice for over a decade.

During one such treatment of Webb, Acer first injected her with anesthetic and then left her to sit for more than an hour. When he finally returned, Webb was crying from intense fear. Acer began the procedure anyway and during the extraction managed to break the tooth off at the gumline. This does occasionally happen but only when the dentist fails to take time to gently, at first, then more forcefully, tease the root loose before attempting to pull it out. Acer apparently did not do this. When the tooth broke, according to Webb, he began digging at the root. Runnells quoted her as saying,

> " While he was sweating and struggling, he described how he was using leverage to dislodge the remaining root...I know there was a lot of bleeding going on in my mouth at that point because he was trying so hard."[10]

After several failed attempts, however, he gave up and instructed Webb to come back for another extraction visit!

"The next day," Runnells wrote, "Acer sent a single rose to Webb, accompanied by a card signed: 'Dr. Acer and Staff.' Acer then billed Cigna [her insurance company] for one flower vase."[10] It is apparent that Acer knew how to stretch his entitlements as well as the limits of ethical dental practice.

Actions Towards Others and the Feedback Filter

Components four and five of the FBI's "motivational model for sexual homicide" concern the outward projection of the killer's inner fantasy life, and the feedback he receives as a result of his sociopathic actions. In adolescence and adulthood,

The murderer's actions become more violent:
assaultive behaviors, burglary, arson, abduction, rape,
nonsexual murder (emphasis added) and finally sexual
murder involving rape, torture, mutilation, and
necrophilia.[8]

Alas! Here was the answer to the dental patient murder riddle. Sexual killers begin their homicidal, fantasy
driven, real life excursions by killing people not for sex,
but purely for dominance, control, revenge and their distorted sense of pleasure.

It is very likely, then, I thought, *had Acer not died of
AIDS when he did, he may have gone on to kill gay sex
partners for the sake of elevated arousal and tension relief.* At once, another terrifying possibility occurred to
me. *Maybe he did kill one or more gay sex partners between 1987 and 1989 before he became really ill.* I wonder if there were any unresolved gay murder cases
pending between Ft. Lauderdale and Stuart?

I went back to the FBI report and continued reading:

First, the early violent acts are reinforced, as the
murderers either are able to express rage without
experiencing negative consequences or are impas-
sive to any prohibitions against these actions. Second, impulsive and erratic behavior discourages
friendships. The failure to make friends leads to
isolation and interferes with the ability to resolve
conflicts, to develop positive empathy, and to control impulses. Furthermore, there is no challenge to
their beliefs that they were entitled to act the way
they do. The men either as children or adolescents
feel estranged from people. Although *that does not
mean that superficially they cannot relate to
people, it does indicate that in terms of socially
effective learning, they have major deficits.* (empha-

sis added) They are loners; they are self-preoccu-
pied. Either by daydreaming or fantasies, they become absorbed in their own thoughts.[8]

Now I could easily understand how it would have
been possible for Acer to have continued to practice dentistry, persuade patients that he was trustworthy, meet
with heterosexual friends for weekly sporting engage-
ments, and carry on some superficial acquaintances—all
without revealing or violating his socially destructive
and sexually prohibited fantasy life.

Regarding the "feedback filter" the report continued,

Given the detailed and repetitive thinking patterns of
these murderers, it is not surprising to learn that the
murderer reacts to and evaluates his actions toward
others and toward himself. These reactions and evaluations influence his future actions...the 'feedback
filter'...feeds back into the killer's patterned responses
and filters his earlier actions into a continued way of
thinking. (In other words)... through the feedback
filter, the murderer's earlier actions are justified, errors are sorted out, and corrections are made to pre-
serve and protect the internal fantasy world and to
avoid restrictions from the external environment.[11]

*The intense attention Acer must have given to his fantasy
world was incredible*, I thought. I was stunned to realize
sexual killers and apparently Acer too preferred this inner
world and go to great lengths to defend it.

One murderer described by the Burgess group of investigators became more excited by his thoughts about
tricking law enforcement agents as time went on. "In this
peculiar evolution of events," they reported, "he now
experienced himself as more involved in the social
world."[11]

The FBI investigators concluded:

In part, psychological models of motivation for sexual murder have focused on models of displacement of rage and frustration from primary caretakers in the lives of sexual murderers. Although these symbolic artifacts may operate, a more direct understanding of the potential for violence and criminal behavior resides in the fantasy life and basic cognitive operations of murderers. A context of justifying socially abhorrent acts provides support for the murderers' aggressive, violent fantasies. This structure, limited to its sensory arousal capacities, maintains and perpetuates the destructive acts.[11]

It was an eye-opener for me to have read this. I too had approached the Acer case analysis from a purely psychological/psychoanalytic perspective. In doing so I was truly limited in being able to fully comprehend the inner dynamics and thinking of Dr. David Acer. *This model is absolutely brilliant!* I thought.

Our motivation model suggests that traumatic and early damaging experiences to the murderers as children set into motion a pattern of cognition (thinking). Although there may be initial attempts to work through the troublesome effects of the experience, attempts to do so become patterns for limiting choices such as aggression being the only method for dealing with conflict. In addition, a structure of thinking that motivates and sustains deviant behavior through developmental and interpersonal failure and through the alliance of distorted perceptions and affect [emotions] begins to emerge. Of particular importance is the activation of aggression and its link with sexual expression. The lack of attachment to others gives a randomness to the sexual crimes; however, scrutiny of the thinking patterns of the offenders indicates that there is planning of the crimes whether they rely on chance encounters with any victim or whether they are planned to snare victims.[12]

Had Acer planned in his isolated fantasy world the real life injection of his dental patients? Was this done to help him resolve his anger—emotional issues principally "linked with sexual expression"—homosexuality, and AIDS along with his desire to assert power, control and revenge over his enemies? Did his alleged selection of mainstream American patients serve a much greater sociopathic purpose: sharing his strife with sexuality, anxiety, and AIDS with everyone in the United States? At this point in the investigation, I believed Parsons. I wondered whether the rest of the world would believe him too.

Table 1. Dental Patients Infected with HIV by Dr. David J. Acer

CDC ID	Name	Age	Profile
A	Kimberly Bergalis	Teenager	College student
B	Barbara Webb	Elderly	Grandmother and school teacher
C	Richard Driscall	Young Adult	Citrus plant foreman
E	Lisa Shoemaker	Young Adult	Undisclosed
G	John Yecs	Young Adult	Undisclosed
H	Sherry Johnson	Adolescent	Grade school student

Table 2. Dr. David Acer's Descriptive Personality Traits

As Reported By Heterosexual and Homosexual Friends, Family, and Acquaintances

Positive Traits	(Source)	Negative Traits	(Source)
Kind	C	Loner/Isolated	C,I
Benevolent	HTA	Deceitful/Compulsive Liar	—
Compassionate	F,M,HTA	Shy/Introverted	C
Sensitive	C	Unremarkable	C
Studious	C	Aggressive when drinking	HMF,HMA
Intelligent	C	Angry	HMF,HMA
Skillful	C	Promiscuous	HMF,HMA
Technically Competent	C	Selfish/Self-Centered	HMF,HMA,I
Independent	M	Sloppy when drunk	HMF,HMA
Scientifically Trained	I	Depressive	—
		Alcoholic	HMF,HMA
		Extremely protective of mother	M,I
		Dependent (on mother)	—
		Extremely defensive about confrontation	HMA,I
		Confused/Misguided	I
		Negligent/Neglectful	HMF,HMA,I
		Sexual Fetishes	HMF,HMA,I
		Secretive	F

Copyright © 1993 Leonard G. Horowitz. All rights reserved.

Source Key: F = Family (Stepfather, Siblings) HMA = Homosexual Acquaintances
M = Mother HTA = Heterosexual Acquaintances
HTF = Heterosexual Friends C = Commonly Observed By Those Who Knew Him
I = CDC & Other Investigators HMF = Homosexual Friend

Table 3. Characteristic Differences Between Organized Versus Disorganized Murderers[†]

Organized	Disorganized
Personal Profile	
• Intelligent, • Skilled in occupation, • Likely to think out and plan the crime, • Likely to be angry and depressed at the time of the murder, • Likely to have a precipitating stress (financial, marital, female, job), • Likely to have a car in decent condition, • Likely to follow crime events in media, and • Likely to change jobs or leave town.	• Be low birth order children, • Come from home w/unstable work for father, • Have been treated with hostility as a child, • Be sexually inhibited and sexually ignorant, and to have sexual aversions, • Have parents w/histories of sexual problems, • Frightened and confused at time of crime, • Know who the victim is, • Live alone, and • Committed the crime closer to home/work.
Crime Scene Profile	
• Plan murders well ahead of time, • Use restraints on their victims, • Commit sexual acts with live victims, • Show or display control of victim (i.e., manipulate, threaten, induce fear), • Use a vehicle,	• Murders not well planned; more spontaneous, • Position dead body, • Perform sexual acts on dead body, • Keep dead body, • Try to depersonalize the body, • Not use a vehicle

Copyright © 1993 Leonard G. Horowitz. All rights reserved.

† Ressler RK, Brugess AW, Douglas JE, Hartman, CR, and D'Agostino, Sexual killers and their victims: Identifying patterns through crime scene analysis". J. Interpersonal Violence 1986;1;3:288-308. In: *Criminal Investigative Analysis: Sexual Homicide.* U.S. Department of Justice Federal Bureau of Investigation, National Center for the Analysis of Violent Crimes, FBI Academy. Quantico, VA 1990.

TABLE 4
Frequency of Reported Behavior Indicators in Adulthood for 28 Sexual Murderers† as Compared with Behavior Patterns of Dr. David Acer As Observed By Family, Friends, and Acquaintances

28 Sexual Murderers		Frequency		Dr. David Acer's Symptoms and Behaviors	
Rating	Behavior	n	(%)	Behavior	Source
1	Assaultive to adults	28	86	Ritual of coming on very strong with gay men after getting drunk	HMF,HMA
2	Daydreaming	27	81	Spent free time in quiet isolation; repetitive tasks at work conducive to daydreaming	C
3	Compulsive masturbation	27	81	Known for sexual fetishes; routinely sought unsuspecting gay men and boys	HMF,HMA,I
4	Isolation	26	73	Loner/isolated; quiet; shy; unremarkable; secretive	C
5	Rebelliousness	25	72	Frequently spoke of CDC and organized medicine with contempt	HMF,HMA
6	Chronic lying	28	68	Chronic lying	C
7	Poor body image	26	62	Poor body image/maintained physical fetish; extremely concerned w/looks	C
8	Stealing	25	56	Provided dental care to maximize revenue rather than serve patient needs	I
9	Nightmares	21	52	Unknown	
10	Sleep problems	22	50	Unknown	
11	Phobias	24	50	Paranoid that mother and "straight" world would find out his sexual preference	C

Source Key: C = Commonly Observed By Those Who Knew Him   HMF = Homosexual Friend   HMA = Homosexual Acquaintances

I = CDC & Other Investigators

† Burgess AW, Hartman, CR, Ressler RK, Douglas JE, and McCormack A. Sexual homicide: A motivational Model. J. Interpersonal Violence 1986;1;3:288-308. In:*Criminal Investigative Analysis: Sexual Homicide.* U.S. Department of Justice Federal Bureau of Investigation, National Center for the Analysis of Violent Crimes, FBI Academy. Quantico, VA 1990.

Table 5. Essentially Identical Match of Personal and Crime Scene Profiles Between 36 Sexual Killers Studied by the FBI[†] and Dr. David Acer

Sexual Homicide Group	Dr. David Acer
Personal Profile	
• Intelligent, • Skilled in occupation, • Likely to think out and plan the crime, • Likely to be angry and depressed at the time of the murder, • Likely to have a precipitating stress (financial, marital, female, job), • Likely to have a car in decent condition, • Likely to follow crime events in media, and • Likely to change jobs or leave town.	• Intelligent and "scientifically educated," • Skilled in occupation, • Likely thought out and planned the crime, • Was just diagnosed with oral KS; angry and depressed at the time of the murder, • Had several precipitating stresses (financial, family, job), • Had a car in decent condition, • Followed crime events on television, and • Knew he would have to stop practicing and die.
Crime Scene Profile	
• Plan murders well ahead of time, • Use restraints on their victims, • Commit sexual acts with live victims, • Show or display control of victim (i.e., manipulate, threaten, induce fear), • Use a vehicle.	• Likely planned murders well ahead of time, • Victims were voluntarily "restrained" in chair • Routinely/compulsively risked transmitting HIV to other gays knowing he had AIDS, • Issues of control, manipulation, perceived threat, and fear inherent in occupation, • Used a vehicle to leave the crime scene.

† Ressler RK, Brugess AW, Douglas JE, Hartman, CR, and D'Agostino, Sexual killers and their victims: Identifying patterns through crime scene analysis". J. Interpersonal Violence 1986;1;3:288-308. In: *Criminal Investigative Analysis: Sexual Homicide.* U.S. Department of Justice Federal Bureau of Investigation, National Center for the Analysis of Violent Crimes, FBI Academy. Quantico, VA 1990.

Table 6. A Comparison of Factors Associated with Individuals Who Knowingly Exposed Others to HIV[†] and Dr. David Acer[*]

Four Reported Cases	Dr. David J. Acer
Critical Observations	
• Black African Americans,	• White Anglo Saxon,
• Gay or bisexual,	• Gay or bisexual,
• Drug dependency background,	• Drug dependency background,
• Lower socio-economic class,	• Middle socio-economic class,
• Found out about HIV status incidentally and did not seem prepared for it,	• Found out about HIV status incidentally and did not seem prepared for it,
• Long period between HIV/AIDS diagnosis and acceptance of the disease as indicated by time of enrollment in service agency,	• Long period between HIV/AIDS diagnosis and acceptance of the disease as indicated by time of enrollment in service agency,
• Lacked social support system and no immediate family support at the time of diagnosis,	• Lacked social support system and no immediate family support at the time of diagnosis,
• Questionable adequacy or consistency of pretest and post test counseling	• Questionable adequacy or consistency of pretest and post test counseling

† Poku KA. Knowingly exposing others to HIV: Four case reports and critique. *AIDS Patient Care* 1992;6:5-10
* Runnells RR. *AIDS In the Dental Office? The Story of Kimberly Bergalis and Dr. David Acer.* Fruit Heights, UT: I.C. Publications, Inc., 1993.

Table 7. Secretaries Appointed by the Governors to Run the Florida HRS During the Acer Case Investigation

Name	Dates of Service
Mr. Greg Coler	February 1987 to December 1990
Mr. Robert Williams (Acting Secretary) (Secretary)	January 1991 to May 1991 May 1991 to March 1993
Lt. Governor Buddy McKay (Acting Secretary)	March 1993 to July 1993
Mr. H. James Towey	July 1993 to present

Source: Florida HRS

Figure 1. A "Motivational Model for Sexual Homicide" Developed by the FBI's Investigating Team of Burgess, Hartman, Ressler, Douglas and McCormack.

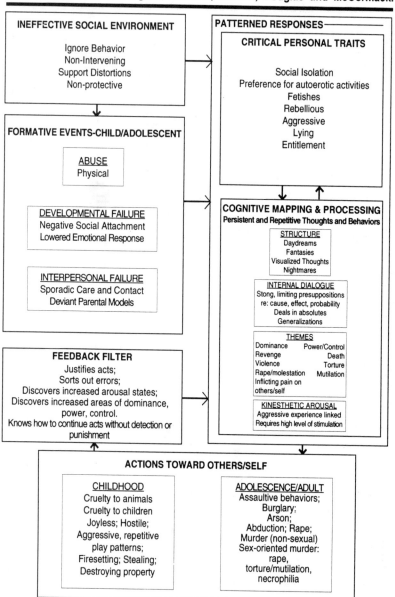

INEFFECTIVE SOCIAL ENVIRONMENT

Ignore Behavior
Non-Intervening
Support Distortions
Non-protective

FORMATIVE EVENTS-CHILD/ADOLESCENT

ABUSE
Physical

DEVELOPMENTAL FAILURE
Negative Social Attachment
Lowered Emotional Response

INTERPERSONAL FAILURE
Sporadic Care and Contact
Deviant Parental Models

FEEDBACK FILTER
Justifies acts;
Sorts out errors;
Discovers increased arousal states;
Discovers increased areas of dominance, power, control.
Knows how to continue acts without detection or punishment

PATTERNED RESPONSES

CRITICAL PERSONAL TRAITS

Social Isolation
Preference for autoerotic activities
Fetishes
Rebellious
Aggressive
Lying
Entitlement

COGNITIVE MAPPING & PROCESSING
Persistent and Repetitive Thoughts and Behaviors

STRUCTURE
Daydreams
Fantasies
Visualized Thoughts
Nightmares

INTERNAL DIALOGUE
Stong, limiting presuppositions
re: cause, effect, probability
Deals in absolutes
Generalizations

THEMES
Dominance   Power/Control
Revenge   Death
Violence   Torture
Rape/molestation   Mutilation
Inflicting pain on
others/self

KINESTHETIC AROUSAL
Aggressive experience linked
Requires high level of stimulation

ACTIONS TOWARD OTHERS/SELF

CHILDHOOD
Cruelty to animals
Cruelty to children
Joyless; Hostile;
Aggressive, repetitive
play patterns;
Firesetting; Stealing;
Destroying property

ADOLESCENCE/ADULT
Assaultive behaviors;
Burglary;
Arson;
Abduction; Rape;
Murder (non-sexual)
Sex-oriented murder:
rape,
torture/mutilation,
necrophilia

Chapter 14.
Matching Acer's Personal and Crime Scene Profiles

Late in the afternoon, Jackie and Alena came home and I ran out to the driveway to greet them.

"You're not going to believe what the FBI sent me!"

"What?"

"A motivational model for sexual homicide which I believe fits Acer to a tee."

"What?"

"Come on in. I'll tell you all about it... How was your day... How did our supermodel fair?"

"Awful!"

"How come?"

"She wouldn't sit still and when they gave her a $20,000 prototype to demo, she threw it across the room and broke it!"

"Oh well, so much for a successful career in baby modeling... O.K. here's the scoop about the FBI report. You're not going to believe this..." The next day I decided to follow up on my hunch Acer may have murdered one or more of the gay men and boys he was known to have solicited. I first called the Stuart police department to ask for help in locating the officer who might be able to give me this answer. I was immediately directed to the Detective Department of the Martin County Sheriff's Office. Upon telephoning, my call was forwarded to their Chief Investigator, Lt. Louis Vaughan.

Detective Vaughan first questioned why I wanted this information. When I mentioned the Acer case and the FBI findings regarding sex-related homicide, he said, "No, we don't have any unresolved homosexual murder cases, but did you know that Lt. Johnnie Johnson, Sherry Johnson's father works here?"

"No," I said, "What a coincidence. I know that Sherry reported to the press that she feels it was murder, and I would be happy to support her testimony if I can be of any help."

"I'll give Lt. Johnson your telephone number," Lt. Vaughan said. We then said goodbye and hung up.

As soon as I hung up the phone, I had a disturbing thought. *I just spilled the beans to the chief detective who's very good friends with Johnnie Johnson. The Johnsons would probably lose their suits against Cigna and CNA if they considered my evidence. That's worth well over a million dollars to them and you can probably buy a hit man for less than $50,000. What am I insane?*

I got up from my desk and consulted Jackie with my concerns.

"You've really got a big mouth," she said. "You've got to be more careful about whom you tell this stuff to."

"You're right."

"But relax, I don't think we have to worry unless they call back to find out just how much we know," Jackie comforted.

With that, I went back to work updating my list of Acer's descriptive personality traits, and comparing these with the personal and crime scene profiles developed by the FBI.

First I reviewed Acer's positive personality traits including: kindness[1,2], benevolence[3], compassion[4], sensitivity and gentleness[5], studiousness and intelligence[6], skill and technical competence[6], shyness and quietness[6,7], independence[6] and scientific training[2].

Next I reassessed his most reported negative traits including: introversion[8], chronic compulsive lying and deceit[8,9,10], preferred and chronic isolation[10,11,12], being unremarkable[6] (i.e, lacking any clear physical or emotional defining features), aggressiveness[10], sloppy and assertive when drunk[13,14], chronic alcoholism[13,14], chronic anger[13], depressive/lethargic[13], fearful of others discovering his homosexuality[2,15], selfish/self-centered[5,16], rebellious regarding the CDC and organized health care for a perceived lack of sensitivity towards AIDS patient care and AIDS research[4,13,14], uncooperative with authorities[17,18] extremely defensive and protective of his mother[19], dependent on his mother[19], confused/misguided[5,7], negligent/neglectful[8,10,20], very secretive[2,21,22], compulsively driven to satisfy his sexual urges (i.e., sexual fetishes)[7,8,10,16,22,23], poor body image (i.e., physical fetishes)[6], lived in denial of personal and public safety concerns[10,20], and entertained himself by watching television[24] (normally a benign behavior, according to Ressler et al., television viewing may correlate with sexual homicidal behavior in that sexual killers most often watch the news on television to reenact the crime in their minds and gain additional pleasure.)[25].

Then I considered the eleven most common symptoms and behaviors Burgess et al. found among sexual killers and compared these with Acer's negative traits (see Table 4). I immediately saw that Acer's negative traits and behaviors matched nine out of the eleven indicators for sexual murderers as established by the FBI. It seemed to me that five of nine matches were strongly related. These included: 1) compulsive sexual fulfillment, 2) isolation, 3) rebelliousness against the CDC, the U.S. Public Health Service, and homophobic society, 4) chronic lying, and 5) poor body image.

It appeared that three more were moderately well related including: 1) the frequent ritual of coming on very strongly and aggressively to gay men after getting intoxicated; 2) spending free time in quiet isolation wherein daydreaming can take place (along with working in a profession wherein repetitive tasks are highly conducive to fantasizing); and 3) a severe paranoia that his mother, patients, and the straight community would find out he was gay.

The final matched factor was that of "stealing." Runnells had documented that Acer would avoid providing low cost dental services, substituting much more expensive work. This, being clearly unethical, I reasoned was close to stealing, the behavior that 56% of the sexual killers acknowledged.

The two other factors present in this FBI profile could not be matched against Acer's personal profile because the behaviors, nightmares and sleep problems, were not socially obvious, and thus were not documented.

I showed this comparative analysis to Jackie and said, "Nine matches and two unknowns out of eleven is pretty close."

"That's incredible," Jackie responded.

I then sat down to do a second cross matching. This one to determine the fit between Acer's personal profile and the model profiles of thirty-six sexual killers developed by a second group of FBI investigators headed by Special Supervisory Agent Robert Ressler.[25] These results are shown in Table 5.

Unreal. I thought. *It's a virtually identical match for all eight of the factors.* "Jackie, come look at this!"

Seconds later Jackie nodded her head in disbelief over what I was showing her.

Next, I cross matched Acer's dental office "crime scene" profile with the Ressler group's crime scene composite. Ressler's team found that:

> Facets of the criminal's personality are evident in his offense... An organized murderer is one who appears to plan his murders and who displays control (e.g., absence of clues) at the crime scene.

As seen in Table 3, the disorganized murderer is less apt to plan, and his crime scenes display haphazard behavior, for instance, the presence of clues at crime scene. In contrast, organized killers left little if any evidence behind for authorities to solve the crime. To help in this investigation process, the Ressler group sought to,

> Identify variables that may be useful in profiling murderers and on which the organized and disorganized murderers differ.[25]

As can be seen by reviewing Table 5, Acer's crime scene profile was essentially indistinguishable from those of organized sexual killers.

Once again, all five of the FBI composite factors could be seen to fit the Acer case exactly.

Speculation or Criminal Investigatory Science?

Ressler's group also noted that isolation is the most consistently reported behavior among sexual killers and that both isolation and sexual homicide is significantly correlated with childhood sexual abuse.[26]

Law enforcement authorities define motiveless-murder as:

> The victim is a stranger and there is no profit to be gained from the death of the victim-suggests that the victim and offense must be seen as having symbolic meaning to the offender reflecting sadistic fantasies.[26]

Furthermore they stated,

> That from an early age, the men had difficulties in both social and sexual relationships. They suggest that this failure in social/sexual approach might be partly responsible for the development of a feeling of inadequacy and lack of assertiveness.[26]

After reading this, I recalled, *Lack of assertiveness was another Acer trait commonly observed by his heterosexual friends and family.*[7,10] I also couldn't help but think, *Maybe his mother's extreme protectiveness and defensiveness was a symptom of a perceived/felt inadequacy or lack of assertiveness on the part of her son.*[6]

The Ressler group went on to report as did the Burgess group, that the killer's childhood trauma(s) and ineffective coping mechanisms lead to sadistic fantasizing in
which the killer in an effort to overcome his insecurities
and social inadequacies, repeatedly expresses his power
and control through imagery, which progressively conditions the need and desire to commit first nonsexual then
sexual crimes in the real world.[27,28]

Their group went on to report that,

Hypersexuality or the sexualization of relationships is
an important indicator of sexually abused children.[26]

Apparently, Acer drank ritually to gain confidence and
become more aggressive.[14] Then he would contentiously
come on to men and boys.[15] Burgess et al.[29] state that
among sexual killers when:

Sexuality is expressed aggressively towards others, it
reflects directly on the aggressive and exploitive nature of the initial abuse.[26]

Ressler et al. went on to speculate that,

The adult role of the abuser in the original childhood victimization is maintained [by the killer] in
the repeated fantasy and thus the preferred sexual
relationship is a *child*/adult pairing.[26]

Could this be why Acer's preference included boys, I questioned?

People Who Intentionally Transmit HIV

Now that I felt most assured that Acer's personality
matched the killer type, I decided to search through back
issues of my scientific journals trying to find a paper
which evaluated people who had been known to have

intentionally infected others with their HIV. After about an hour of searching, I struck pay dirt. In a back issue of *AIDS Patient Care*, Dr. Kwabena Poku an assistant professor in the Department of Psychiatry and Behavioral Sciences at Meharry Medical College in Nashville reported on an evaluation he had performed on four other HIV-positive people who knowingly exposed others to their virus.[30]

Poku reported that "abrupt and abbreviated" pre-test counseling was one of the most common findings among the individuals who knowingly risked other people's lives. In addition to this, Dr. Poku noted that:

> Learning about their seropositivity was associated with certain types of psychological distress symptoms such as anxiety, anger, depression, sexual dysfunction, and other untoward effects such as increased illicit drug use and disruption of relationships. It is postulated that the abruptness of the message about HIV seropositivity and AIDS might have been (predisposing) factors for the subject's behavior. They seemed to have been shocked into erratic compulsive behaviors.[30]

In all, Poku listed eight critical observations made of his group of people who knowingly spread the AIDS virus to others. These included:

• All clients were black.

• All clients had gay/bisexual relationships.

• All subjects had drug dependency backgrounds.

• All subjects were within the lower socio-economic class based on education and job history.

- All subjects found out about their HIV seropositive status incidentally and did not seem prepared for it.

- Long periods elapsed between HIV/AIDS diagnosis and acceptance of the disease as indicated by time of enrollment in an HIV/AIDS service agency.

- All seemed to lack a social support system and there was no immediate family support at the time of diagnosis.

- Adequacy and consistency of pre-test and post-test counseling for the clients are questionable.[30]

As shown in Table 6, besides the fact that David Acer was white and established in the middle class, he maintained all the other factors associated with Poku's study group.

Legal, Ethical, Moral and Financial Concerns

After documenting the evidence I felt adequately settled the murder/accident debate once and for all, I prepared two papers for submission to professional journals. The first article, submitted to the *Journal of the American Medical Association (JAMA)*, presented and discussed the match between Acer's personal and crime scene profiles and those of thirty six sexual killers. The other, critically reviewed the CDC report and apparent HRS and CDC conspiracy to cover-up the facts. This I submitted to the *Journal of the American Dental Association (JADA)*. I spoke with both editors prior to submitting the papers, and informed each about the need for their reviewers to reference the FBI reports, which I sent a copy of, as well as Runnells's book. I also informed *JADA* about my concern regarding the possible repercussions of someone at the HRS/CDC finding out about my discoveries before the information was released to the press. I requested that he not send the paper out for review to anyone who had dental public health connections for obvious reasons.

Because my family and I alone would have to live with the risk, anxiety, and responsibility of having this information until it was made public, I considered every option about how to release it most intelligently, professionally, and quickly. The fact that professional organizations discourage releasing information to the press prior to a report's thorough review and acceptance created additional pressure. I felt torn between my desire for safety; my concerns about someone stealing my work and then representing it as their own, and my desire for gaining financial remuneration for my long and hard work, versus the professional/scientific route of waiting patiently for the paper's acceptance—often a period of months.

After many sleepless nights, Jackie reminded me, "It's foolish to worry about it. You're only hurting yourself. Just get to work on your book."

Soon thereafter, I ran into a patient and friend of mine, Martha, who encouraged me to contact an attorney in Boston whom she thought could help me produce a screenplay as well as provide legal advice. A week later, I met with the lawyer and discussed my findings. He immediately encouraged me to contact CIGNA and CNA, the two insurance companies who had been settling out of court with Acer's victims. He told me the information I had would probably save them millions of dollars since they would not have to pay if it was shown that Acer was a murderer and not just negligent. He suggested that perhaps the HRS would be liable for damages, though the case would be hard to litigate.

The next day, I considered the ethical, moral, social, and financial values of following the attorney's advice. After carefully weighing the pros and cons of the decision, including the ramifications for the victims and their families—the probability that they would likely have to sue the HRS rather than CIGNA and CNA, I decided to rely on my lifelong philosophy, "the truth always works."

I contacted the attorneys for the two insurance companies. I informed them that I was able to provide substantial evidence that Acer intentionally infected his patients and that if they were interested in saving several million dollars in future claims, they should get back to my attorney. Much to my amazement, they never called back.

For weeks I thought, *Maybe they preferred to settle out of court rather than receive the negative publicity which would likely result from a long drawn-out litigation process.* I would soon realize another frightening possibility—one that was infinitely more unjust.

Chapter 15.
The HRS, Reno
and Clinton Connection

As I awaited a response from the scientific journals and worked feverishly on this book, what continued to hold my fascination was the interesting comment made by GAO investigators in their official report:

> Because the personnel at the CDC and HRS are health investigators, not criminal investigators, *they* (italics added) brought this matter to the attention of the attorney general in Florida.[1]

I spent months wondering who "they" were, and despite knowledge that Parson's testimony centered on Acer's homicidal motives, "they" allegedly, according to the GAO report, sent one or more HRS officials to interview Parsons.

But that doesn't make sense, I thought, *the HRS investigators are public health personnel, not criminal detectives. They would have been incapable of evaluating Parson's criminal evidence!*

I sat perplexed for a minute then considered who at the HRS might have interviewed Parsons or evaluated his testimony? *Surely, the director of the HRS would have been involved since this was undoubtedly the most important AIDS and infection control case in the history of American medicine.*

I had called the HRS and was informed that there were several HRS secretaries (directors) between 1987 to the present. The Secretaries or Acting Secretaries (listed in Table 7) were appointed by two Governors during the Acer case investigation. All but Greg Coler were appointed by Governor Lawton Chiles. I knew from the way I had been previously rebuffed when I called the HRS, I would not be able to find out who was involved in the investigation. I also thought that if "they" knew I was investigating them, my life and perhaps the lives of Jackie and the baby could also be in jeopardy.

My uneasiness stemmed from the stories my father told and what I had learned myself by reading the newspapers. I knew the difference between organized crime and politics as usual, was often indistinguishable. One case, in my hometown, had led to the killing of an FBI agent who's death was made to look like a suicide. *People have been killed for much less than what I was about to disclose with this book*, I thought. Alleging a conspiracy by politicians and government health officials to cover-up the truth about a case costing tens of thousands of American's lives, and increased burnout and dropout among health professionals—was very risky. I tried not to think about it.

On August, 28, 1993, my best friend from dental school, invited Jackie, Alena and I to their annual cook-out. When we arrived, we were immediately greeted by my friend and another mutual acquaintance, Greg, whom I hadn't seen in several years. As I began to share my research about the Acer case, our mutual friend began disclosing highly controversial information about the Florida HRS.

Most incredible, he said, "I think, Janet Reno, the Attorney General, had been assigned to investigate the HRS during the time you say Acer was being investigated."

"What! Wait a minute," I said, "How do you know all this about the HRS?"

"My first cousin is very active in Florida politics and 'family rights'. I know he's been investigating the HRS for fraud and misconduct on many levels."

"You've got to be kidding!" *What a coincidence*, I thought, *I can't believe I'm hearing this.*

"Not only that," he said, "I understand that Hillary Clinton is a good friend of Janet Reno, and that the two of them had worked closely together in advocating children's rights programs in the state. My cousin can tell you a lot more about it, but he takes the position that these new laws really infringe on the civil rights of families."

"Can you give me your cousin's name and telephone number, I'd love to talk with him."

"Sure, I'll call you with it early this week."

On the way home that night, my uneasiness turned into full-blown paranoia. Jackie was off swimming with Alena during the entire conversation I had with Greg, so when I said, "Now, I'm really paranoid." She didn't know why.

"How come?"

"There's a good possibility our investigation might lead to evidence involving the newly appointed Attorney General of the United States—Janet Reno."

During the drive home, I explained the details of my conversation with Greg, and Jackie became equally concerned.

The Family Rights Investigation

I never really knew how deep paranoia can strike until the following day when our telephones began to malfunction.

"Don't you hate it when people call, then hang up just when you pick up the phone?"

Jackie nodded.

After two similar occurrences over the next twenty minutes I cautiously announced, "Jack, I think our phones are being tapped."

Our conversations about the Acer investigation soon turned to cautious whispers.

By mid-week, unable to stand the suspense of waiting any longer for Greg's call, I called him. He apologized for not getting back to me sooner and retrieved his cousin's phone number. I immediately placed the call to Mr. John Ostalkiewicz.

Ostalkiewicz's wife answered the telephone and told me that, "John is volunteering at the Family Rights Committee office in Orlando. Would you like that number?"

"Sure."

About fifteen minutes after leaving a message on their answering machine, my call was returned.

Mr. Paul Gordon, the Manager of the Family Rights Committee, Inc. told me that John had just stepped out of the office for a short time, and asked what the call was in reference to. I explained my investigation and what John's cousin had told me about the Florida HRS.

Mr. Gordon confirmed the allegations and said that their organization had been battling the HRS for several years. "We literally have thousands of documents which support allegations of political corruption and social wrongdoing by them," he said. "John, however, is the Chairman of Family Rights, and he's most knowledgeable. I'm sure he can fill you in on the details."

That afternoon, John called me back, and we spent about twenty minutes discussing our different HRS investigations. John had been investigating them primarily due to their enforcement of "child advocacy" laws which both Janet Reno and Hillary Rodham Clinton had championed in Florida and elsewhere.

"The HRS is the largest state agency in the United States with an annual budget of over $9 billion," John reported. "They have more than 40,000 employees and are one of the most corrupt state bureaucracies in America. They get away with it because the only people that investigate them are people within the HRS. They have a long record of violating family rights. They've taken tens of thousands of infants and children away from their parents over the past year and a half; most often without good cause. They label the parents as child abusers and pronounce them guilty before proven innocent. The parents are then put through the ringer—sometimes they lose their jobs—and all have to go to court to prove their innocence. Its a huge racket—the judges in the abuse courts, their lawyers, and their counselors are all making money for the HRS and the politicians. They have doctors who lie and falsify medical documents too. The parents often spend months and even years fighting losing battles in court to try to get their kids back. In the meantime their families fall apart. It costs many of them over $50,000 before it's all done—and the kids get scarred for life."

"The Family Rights Committee has about 10,000 files we've collected over the past five years documenting all of this," John continued. We have charged them with routinely falsifying legal documents, perjury, and kidnapping... They have agents who are like the secret police. They interrogate people without warrants, and without cause throw many innocent people in jail... Rather than prosecuting hardened criminals, they lure them into counseling too. They are in the counseling business. They get more than $100 dollars an hour for counseling second, third and forth time criminal offenders who they let back out on the street, while prosecuting and jailing many innocent parents alleged to have committed child abuse. You would not believe what's happening down here."

I listened in amazement as John shared his knowledge of the HRS, and after telling him what I knew about the Acer investigation he said, "That doesn't surprise me one bit."

"Do you know who was in charge of the HRS when Acer was first investigated to the time that Bergalis reported he infected her—say from 1987 through 1991 or 92?"

"I believe Greg Coler; he was forced to resign by Lawton Chiles in 1991 because HRS was in such a mess. Chiles then appointed Janet Reno to head a special committee overseeing the HRS commissioned to evaluate and restructure the entire organization," John said. "I can't remember whether Chiles made her director over Bob Williams, or not. I'll have to check our records, and get back to you with the specifics," he concluded.

"That would be just great," I responded, "Send me anything else you think I might be interested in reading for my book. I really appreciate your help."

"No problem," John said, "We're happy to do it. After you receive the materials, let me know if I can be of any further assistance."

As I hung up the telephone, I realized that the political embarrassment the HRS would suffer from their admission of having not thoroughly investigated Acer, might have been directed at Janet Reno or Governor Chiles as well. *Now it really begins to make sense,* I thought. *With Reno charged with overseeing the entire HRS, plus her close ties to Hillary Clinton, no wonder they felt an urgent need to cover-up the mess of the Acer investigation, particularly if the HRS was so corrupt.*

The next morning I received a telephone call from an associate producer for an NBC News magazine show. She informed me that her father, a dentist, had taken my "Dentistry in the Age of AIDS" course several months earlier and had recently told her what I had shared about the Acer case. She said she wanted to do a segment emphasizing the irrational fear response of the public to what was reported by the media, and she wanted to schedule me immediately for an interview. I had to decline.

"I don't understand," she said.

"I'm sorry, I'd really love to do the show, but I'm just not ready to release all the information I have just yet," I responded.

"What are you waiting for?" she queried.

"I've got two scientific papers currently being reviewed by JAMA and JADA, I'm just finishing up with my book, and I'm not prepared to speak to the press until one of the papers are accepted or I have my book in print," I explained.

She was very persistent in trying to get me to share what I knew about the Acer case and the CDC's investigation, but after about a half-an-hour of politely declining to offer her what she wanted to hear, she said, "When can we schedule you then?"

"I'd say about in about seven to ten weeks," I said.

"Fine, then I will be in touch and I'm really looking forward to working with you," she concluded.

Background Search on the Reno-Clinton Connection

Rather than sitting around, nervously awaiting the information from the Family Rights Committee, I drove to the local college library to search through back issues of the *New York Times* to see what I could learn about the Reno-Clinton connection. I also wondered whether the HRS had been mentioned during the Attorney General's confirmation hearings.

The first article I found dated back to February, 10, 1993. Reno was being considered for the job by the Clinton Administration. The article stated:

> Ms. Reno is unlike the two other women recently put forward... for the job of the nation's chief law-enforcement officer, in that she has significant experience in the field. She has been the chief prosecu-

tor in the high-crime district of Dade County, which includes Miami, since 1978, and is regarded as a forceful advocate of law enforcement.

. . . Mr Clinton has seen Zoe Baird, a corporate lawyer, and Judge Kimba M. Wood of Federal District Court in New York fall victim to disclosures about their hiring of household help to care for their children.

Ms. Reno, who is single, has no children.[2]

Given her "significant experience in the field" and position as chief prosecutor in a high crime district for almost fifteen years, I thought, if Reno had been overseeing the HRS at the time of the Acer investigation, and had she been around when Acer's medical history or Parsons's deposition was being considered, surely someone as experienced as she would have suspected homicide.

Two days later Reno's selection was announced by an upbeat President who said he "had a high regard for Ms. Reno," and knew of her "through his brother-in-law, Hugh Rodham, a public defender in Miami." Again Mr. Clinton said in support of Reno, ". . . you couldn't be a state's attorney in Dade County for 15 years without having enormous exposure to a wide range of issues that the Justice Department deals with."[3] Again, I thought, *What about sexual homicide cases?*

The article continued:

She is perhaps best known for her office's prosecution of William Lozano, a police officer charged with killing two black motorists in 1989 in a case that touched off rioting in Miami. The conviction was later overturned.

Ms. Reno has also vigorously prosecuted child abuse cases and been a forceful advocate for children's rights, an important cause of Hillary Rodham Clinton.

Mrs. Clinton had been pressing for a woman to be named Attorney General, and the President said his wife, "knew her and liked her a lot."[3]

After reading this I realized that what John had been saying was on-the-level. It seemed odd that she was best known for prosecuting a killer whose conviction she couldn't successfully defend. Moreover, here was documentation that she and the First Lady had been friends and mutual supporters of the "children's rights" movement John and the Family Rights Committee had been fighting against.

The article also said:

Minutes after Judge Wood's candidacy was scuttled, White House officials said, they placed a call to Ms. Reno to set up an appointment with her and Mr. Clinton. The officials said that at that time, Ms. Reno had already been through an initial background check of her public records... Officials said private lawyers began reviewing her personal documents Wednesday morning and completed the process on Thursday...

White House officials said they were absolutely certain that Ms. Reno had no problem with hiring illegal immigrants or not paying taxes on household help.

"We asked much more pointed questions this time around," said an aide closely involved in the review process. "Who have you hired as domestic help? Who have you hired as a nanny? Have you ever hired any other helping hands? We were trying to cover all the bases."[3]

Trying to cover all the bases, I questioned? *Given her lack of children and her powerful position of overseeing HRS activities at the time of the Acer investigation, more appropriate questions would have been, "What do you know about the bungling of the Dr. David Acer Florida case investigation by the HRS and CDC?" or if John was right, "What do you know about the allegations of child abuse and kidnapping being lodged against the HRS?"*

Finally, after ticking off Reno's accomplishments, the President made it a point to acknowledge her integrity.

> I want to say to you that everyone I know who knows and has worked with Janet agrees that she possesses one quality most essential to being Attorney General—unquestioned integrity," the President said. "She demonstrated throughout her career a commitment to principles that I want to see enshrined at the Justice Department. No one is above the law."[3]

As I read this I wondered whether the President's statement, "No one is above the law" would apply for those directly involved in the decision to sacrifice the truth along with tens of thousands of lives and the American people's confidence in health care—even if it might have involved the Florida Attorney General, the Governor, and the person Clinton was speaking about?

In another article, written by Larry Rohter of the *New York Times,* adjacent the one cited above, opposition to the Reno nomination was voiced by police organizations and others who argued:

> She is not tough enough on crime or criminals. In particular, she has drawn fire for once having declared, "My highest priority is to protect the rights of the guilty, not to convict the guilty."

Many Miami lawyers and judges, though, have accused Ms. Reno of not being aggressive enough in
pursuing big, tough cases, especially those involving police and public officials.

In recent years, the State Attorney's office here has
deferred to Federal prosecutors in several big corruption cases.[4]

*If this is so, I considered, it might explain why, if she
was in the powerful position of evaluating and restructuring the operations of the HRS, or involved with the
organization in making decisions about the investigation, she may have turned her back on the whole affair.
This would have fit the pattern of avoiding politically
sensitive cases, and/or the corruption that John
Ostalkiewicz alleged exists at the HRS.*

The article also stated:

The only outright opposition to Ms. Reno's nomination has come from conservative Republicans and
some Christian religious organizations. They argue,
among other things, that she has been soft on pornography, failed to curb crime and is, in the words
of Anthony R. Martin, a Republican candidate for
Governor, "a high priestess of political correct-
ness..."[4]

The following Tuesday, February 16, 1993, another
interesting article by Rohter appeared in the *New York
Times* which described some of Reno's professional behaviors. The article began by stating:

Among the lawyers and investigators who have
worked for her, State Attorney Janet Reno of Dade
County has always inspired a certain dread with a
little black book she keeps. In it... a detailed record
of the progress—or lack thereof—in every case that
interests her.

"Everybody hated that little black book," said Wayne
Black, one of Ms. Reno's former investigators. "She
would ask you to brief her, and then two or three
weeks later she'd call you in and refer to the black
book and what you had told her you would be doing.
She was very big into checking up."[5]

I thought, *If this indicates her level of investigative prowess
and administrative competence, had she have taken a personal
interest in this case, then she probably made note of it in her "little
black book" along with detailed records on the case's progress.*

Further suggestion of her possible involvement in the
investigation stated by Jose Quinon, a former assistant
state attorney now in private practice in Miami. He
stated:

" No matter how much she has to adjust, I'm sure
she will keep a pretty strong hand on things and
will definitely demand to be made aware of every
important decision... She's a hands-on type of person, no matter what the type of system or the number of individuals she will be supervising. She has a
need to control things."[5]

Rohter's article continued:

When a case involved an issue in which Ms. Reno
took a personal interest, she often bypassed supervisors and went directly to those in the field. "I predict here and now that if she hears about some hot
case in some district somewhere, the U.S. Attorney
there will get a call." Mr. Black said with a laugh.
"That's just her management style."[5]

*Given the fact that the entire medical scientific com-
munity was attacking the credibility of the HRS and its
investigation of the Acer case at the exact time Reno was
charged with overseeing the workings of the organization, it is
possible she took an active interest in the case,* I thought. *After*

all, this wasn't just "some hot case."—this was one of the hottest cases in the history of American medicine. Who wouldn't have taken an active interest! Just about everyone in America plus millions more throughout the world were interested in what happened between Acer and his victims. It's hard to imagine that Reno would not have taken a "special interest" in it also, particularly since she had close ties to the Attorney General's office.

If Reno had known of Parsons, I thought, with her "hands-on" management style, she might have gone directly to "those in the field" who the GAO report said interviewed Parsons. If she had, then the critics who believed the CDC and HRS did not have the criminal investigative personnel to thoroughly evaluate the homicidal evidence were wrong.

Was it possible that Reno's expertise was immediately available to HRS officials as well as CDC and Florida Attorney General's office investigators at the time when Jaffe told reporters the CDC may ask for a criminal investigation? Might Reno's presence explain why according to the GAO report, the HRS was directed to conduct the criminal inquiry and investigative interview of Parsons after both the HRS and Attorney General's office acknowledged the need to investigate Parson's homicidal allegations further? I questioned.

I continued my mental probe, Had Reno learned that Dr. Witte, the principal investigator for the HRS and CDC, chose to delete, from the January 18, 1991 MMWR on the Acer investigation, evidence that would draw attention to Acer as a murder suspect—his complete medical history including the use of an alias, falsifying medical documents, lying, deceit, alcoholism, intense sexual promiscuity, physical fetishes, depression, denial, and anger?

It's inexcusable how and why all the criminal evidence got pushed-aside, and entirely deleted from all four official investigation reports. There had to have been clear intent on the part of the HRS, CDC and Florida State Attorney General's office executives to do this. Thus it occurred to me, *had Reno been involved with the HRS during this critical time, then she either didn't become involved, purposely looked the other way, and/or was directly involved in the conspiracy to cover-up the truth about the case.*

I can't imagine, if she was commissioned to evaluate how the HRS was working with her "hands-on" style, close follow up with subordinates, and special attention to the most interesting cases, why this case wasn't solved long ago? I'd sure love to get my hands on her little black book, I thought.

Additionally, Mr. Al Cotera, head of the Miami Fraternal Order of Police said of Ms. Reno:

> I think she is very strong on civil rights... She holds law enforcement to a higher level than the average citizen in her scrutiny of cases... she has always stressed the importance of collaboration in developing a case... She has always believed in working hand in glove with the Federal authorities, and has conducted many investigations on a joint basis.[5]

I wondered, *If this is true, she might have also been overseeing the way in which the HRS collaborated with the CDC on this historic case.*

Finally, the article stated:

> Although the 54-year-old prosecutor has set strict standards of accountability, she also tends to delegate a great deal of authority to subordinates, even those who are young and relatively inexperienced.[5]

Undoubtedly, I thought, *this is what would be claimed by the U.S. Attorney General in the event this and future investigations were to implicate her office in the failed investigation and obvious cover-up. But the fact that she maintained a "little black book" and was a "hands-on type of person" might make it difficult to use this excuse.*

Additional articles about Ms. Reno appeared in the *New York Times* on Friday, February 19, 1993, and then again on Tuesday, March, 9 1993. They discussed the diversion of first time drug offenders and non-career criminals into treatment programs run by the Dade County Court and the county's Department of Human Resources. Judge Stanley Goldstein who ran the Diversion and Treatment Program said:

> The program, the first of its kind, could not operate without the strong support of the Dade County State Attorney, Janet Reno, whom President Clinton has chosen to be Attorney General.

> Ms. Reno, in fact, suggested that the program should have its own courtroom, and that is where a brother of Hillary Rodham Clinton, Hugh Rodham, works as a public defender.[6]

As Mr. Fernandez, Ms. Reno's prosecutor, explained:

> " A lot of people here start using (drugs) again, but they get second, third and fourth chances from the judge. She has told us to let the judge and the treatment people do their jobs and recognized that it is expected that there will be relapses. I basically am here to keep things from getting out of control with career criminals and those with violent crimes."[6]

When I first began reading and considered the concept of diversion of first time drug offenders into educational and behavioral treatment programs this made good sense to me. But when I read Mr. Fernandez's comments a red flag went up. Third and fourth offenses said to me that either the counselors weren't doing a very good job, the selection of offenders was poor, or both.

This story along with the other article published on March 9, further discussed the opposition to Ms. Reno's nomination on the basis that she and her office had been too soft on crime. The allegations by John Ostalkiewicz from the Family Rights Committee about the HRS being in the counseling business was being supported by what I was now reading.

Larry Rohter of the *New York Times* wrote:

> While Ms. Reno has won wide popular support here, winning re-election handily, she has also attracted criticism locally, especially from police officers and some lawyers. Kenneth Harms, who was Chief of the Miami Police Department from 1978 until he was dismissed in an unrelated political dispute in 1984, called Ms. Reno's performance on crime matters seriously deficient.
>
> "She's a very good politician," said Mr. Harms, who is now a private law-enforcement consultant here. "But in terms of putting bad guys in jail, I'm not at all comfortable with her record. The bottom line is that there are too many damn criminals out on the street."... [7]

News of Attorney General Reno's breeze through her confirmation hearings was published the next day in the *New York Times*.[8]

Two weeks later on March 24, 1993 Reno's first major Clinton Administration chore was to dispense of political trouble-makers left over from the Bush Administration including Mr. Jay B. Stephens, the United States Attorney for the District of Columbia. Stephens had reported that he was within one month of making a "critical decision" in his investigation of the powerful House Ways and Means Committee Chairman, Dan Rostenkowski; a Democratic Representative from Illinois and long time Clinton supporter. The *New York Times* article said that "Ms. Reno's order accelerated what had been expected to be a leisurely changeover."

Why was she in such a hurry to get rid of him? I thought.

Reporter David Johnston wrote:

All 93 United States Attorneys knew they would be asked to step down, since all are Republican hold-overs, and 16 have resigned so far. But *the process generally takes much longer and had usually been carried out without the involvement of the Attorney General.*

Ms. Reno is under pressure to assert her control over the appointments at the Justice Department... It was unclear whether Ms. Reno initiated the request for resignations or whether it was pressed on her by the White House. The Attorney General said it was a "joint decision."

Ms. Reno also said she had not decided whether to replace William S. Sessions, the Director of the Federal Bureau of Investigation, who has been found to have violated ethics rules.[8]

That night between Alena's crying, and the stream of thoughts running through my head, I had great difficulty getting any sleep. I kept thinking about what Ostalkiewicz had said about Reno's connection to the HRS, labored over the fact that *not one New York Times reporter* made mention of any association between her and the alleged most corrupt state agency in America. I thought, *Maybe this family rights guy doesn't have his facts straight? Maybe it's best to stop the investigation here and go to press with the information I already have?*

In the morning, Jackie and I decided it was probably best to try to insulate ourselves from harm, and insure the truth about the Acer case would ultimately be spoken. For these reasons, Jackie copied and distributed my two research reports along with earlier copies of this manuscript to several friends throughout New England with the instructions to forward the information to reporters throughout the country in the event something were to happen to our family.

Late in the afternoon, and then again for the next two days I fielded calls from the same NBC News producer requesting additional facts about the case and urging me to go on their show at once. On Saturday morning she telephoned to warn me that Barbara Walters had announced on ABC's *20/20* the night before, that next week she would be interviewing a new witness who would be revealing new facts about the Acer case which would prove it was murder.

"Now will you come on?" she said, "You could lose everything if someone beats you to the punch."

Although, I knew her statement was a Freudian projection expressing her vulnerability about not being the first to air this history making story, her comments still threw me for a loop.

"Look, let me tell you something," I said. "There's just no way that any witness could have put all the pieces of this puzzle together. I suspect she will be interviewing Ed Parsons, but even if there is someone else, I can tell you that the story of Dr. David Acer is just one part of one of the most amazing and incredible true crime tales that could never be imagined. I don't think I have to worry, but thanks for the call."

After I hung up I discussed the situation with my wife and a friend who was visiting. Our friend urged us not to worry and reminded us that the call was typical of a news reporter who was trying to capture a big story. Still, we spent the day and a good part of the evening battling the insecurity within us.

The Big Picture

The next morning seemed to promise a clearer and brighter day. The wind and rain which had dominated the weather, and the fear and depression which had overshadowed our certainty, for the previous two days, was suddenly gone. Jackie and I, with Alena on my back in her backpack, took our usual Sunday morning hike into town for exercise and breakfast.

Along the shore by Back Beach, we ran into a very old friend whom I hadn't seen in about thirty years. He told me he was living in Florida and managed an Eckerd Drugstore which is part of a large chain operating in the Southeastern part of the country. I shared with him what I knew about Acer, and he shared with me what he knew about the HRS.

My friend, who wished to remain anonymous, explained that there were many big changes happening in Florida as a result of a push to implement a state health care program. He mentioned that Eckerd and Walgreens the two principal players in the consumer drug market were in the process of negotiating a deal to become the selected providers of medicines for everyone in the state.

He said, "The Eckerd and Walgreen chains are vying to buy out all the independent and smaller chains. You would not believe the amount of building that's going on too. Eckerd stores are being built all over the place in an effort to position the company for the changes and to meet the demand."

"What's happening to the little guy—the independently owned drugstores?" I asked.

"They're all being bought out or driven out by the chains. After all, most of our money is collected now from third parties—insurance carriers. All of these companies are also making deals with the HRS to be a part of the state run plan."

"Do you think it will really save people money?" I questioned.

"I seriously doubt it," he said, "God knows, our prices aren't exceptionally low. I think a lot of our competitors have lower prices, and apparently, friendlier service based on some of the feedback we've been receiving from our customers." He continued, "We're in the process of making a lot of changes as a company. We've been making money but we're still trying to cut costs by laying off personnel and cutting back on everything from employee bonuses to charitable contributions. We no longer donate to local police departments or the Chamber of Commerce. The only money the company is now giving away is for "EckPac" to support our political action efforts. Everyone is currently making deals to try to get into the system—the hospitals, HMOs and insurance companies are particularly concerned."

The thought, *That's probably why the insurance companies didn't get back to my attorney,* flashed through my mind. *They weren't interested in receiving the evidence that could save them a few million dollars when what I was offering could risk the relationship they had established with the HRS and the chance of making billions of dollars from the HRS's state run health care system.*

After a few more minutes spent discussing the incumbent changes in the HRS's health care monopoly, my friend mentioned that Governor Lawton Chiles was the principal force behind the movement. At that instant, I recalled, what Ostalkiewicz had said about Governor Chiles appointing Janet Reno to head the HRS during the time of the Acer investigation. Then I remembered quickly scanning and copying a *New York Times* article about Chiles and the Florida health care reform program when I was searching for information about Reno.

I thanked my friend for the information, and told him to watch out for his contribution in my upcoming book.

"That's the big picture," I said to Jackie as we continued our walk back to the house.

"What is?" she asked.

"That's why it was so important to keep the HRS free from negative publicity about the Acer case and investigation," I answered.

"I still don't get what you mean," she said.

"Wait a few minutes," I responded, "You'll see when we get home."

On the way back, Jackie and I discussed the incredible series of "coincidences" which consistently brought our investigation to its next level. Every time I thought the investigation was complete, I connected with just the right person who would lead me to take another step towards understanding the big picture. Confident this guidance was being directed by a higher power, we decided to set aside all remaining fear.

Minutes later I retrieved the *New York Times* article I had set aside in a separate file and the two of us sat down to read it. "Florida Blazes Trail to a New Health-Care System" read the title. The article was published on April 4, 1993, about three weeks after Janet Reno had been confirmed as Attorney General. It described how Governor Chiles had stonewalled the Florida legislature, keeping them in session to the wee hours of the morning in order to get them to pass his bill. Larry Rohter wrote:

> Tallahassee, FLA, April 3—The Florida Legislature approved a sweeping overhaul of the state's overburdened health-care system early today, making Florida the first state in the nation to combine free market competition and government regulation in a way similar to the Clinton Administration's plans for controlling soaring medical costs.

> . . . Mr Chiles said he hoped that "Florida's embrace of a system of managed competition, in which large numbers of people and businesses buy health care from organized networks of doctors and hospitals, would be a model for other states as well as to chart the way for the Federal Government," he said.

> . . . In part, Florida's lawmakers were pushed to act by soaring health care spending, which rose to $38 billion last year from $9.4 billion in 1980.

> Phalanx of lobbyists representing hospitals, insurance, companies, doctors, drug manufacturers, pharmacists, malpractice lawyers, laboratories and other special interests watched the creation of 11 Community Health Purchasing Alliances. As envisioned by Mr. Chiles, these new state chartered

regional cooperatives will help employers obtain the best care at the cheapest price and decide what kind of care plans can be offered on the market.

"I don't think there will be immediate savings," Mr. Chiles, a democrat, said shortly after the State Senate passed the package at 1 A.M. today. "But I do think there will be people getting health care who never had a chance to get it before, and there will be small businesses that will be able to cover their people that they were not able to cover before."[9]

"That's what it was all about," I said.

Jackie could only shake her head in disbelief.

"There are now eleven district HRS offices that will control a Florida health care industry grossing well in excess of $38 billion—the archetype for the Clinton administration, to show what they will do to improve the American social welfare, criminal justice, and health care systems."

"No wonder the Clintons chose Reno to come to Washington."

"She had done her job in Florida," I said. "I don't know how long they've been working on it, but it looks to me like Hillary Clinton, Lawton Chiles, Reno and other political cronies, seized control over Florida's social welfare, judicial, law enforcement, and health care agencies. Now that Florida is like a socialistic state, and they took control of its multi-billion dollar conglomerate, the HRS— she gets assigned to the next big job—help do the same for the entire country."

"You're right," Jackie responded. "And if you remember back to Clinton's election, there was all that talk about him needing Florida to win."

"Oh right!" I said, "She and Chiles were critical Clinton supporters. They, in effect, delivered him the Presidency."

Chapter 16:
The Family and
Children's Rights Agendas

Two days later, a big package arrived at the expense of Paul Gordon and the Family Rights Committee, Inc. It contained a book entitled: *The Child Abuse Industry: Outrageous Facts About Child Abuse & Everyday Rebellions Against a System that Threatens Every North American Family*, by Mary Pride, several audiotapes of interviews with parents who had been victimized by the HRS including the hideous details about their struggles to regain their right to see their children and have a family again, and dozens of articles published by national and local newspapers documenting everything that John Ostalkiewicz had told me over the telephone.

I sat and read that, indeed, Janet Reno had been appointed by Lawton Chiles to two important HRS-defining positions. According to an Associated Press report issued as a public relations announcement from Tallahassee on Tuesday January 8, 1991, that is, *immediately* upon Chiles taking over as governor, Janet Reno became head of a special political advisory panel charged with "overseeing the Department of Health and Rehabilitative Services." The article, which appeared in the *Orlando Sentinel*, entitled "HRS can't do everything for everybody, task group's chief says" quoted Reno as saying:

> " We've got limited dollars... Let us recognize that HRS cannot be everything to everybody. Let us recognize that HRS simply cannot substitute for an

American family that has disintegrated and for
American neighborhoods and communities that have
disintegrated."[1]

Now I've always considered myself a liberal Democrat with relatively conservative views about family and
humanistic views about people. When I read this I found
myself agreeing with Reno's position. I did, however,
find it odd that she would be declaring the HRS destitute
given my knowledge that their annual budget was then
about $30 billion. But more peculiar than this was the
fact that she had just been appointed to begin an unbiased investigation of the HRS, and already she was defending it. *She already had a previously defined agenda*, I
thought, *and no intention of conducting an objective investigation into the failings of the HRS.*

Then she went on to say:

" And to knock HRS around the head for every
tragedy that occurs because some other much more
long-standing institution has failed is not right."[1]

I balked when I read this as I realized she was attacking the "institution" of family. I re-read the February 12,
1993 *New York Times* article by Larry Rohter which described Reno's family life. Numerous references were
made to her mother's influence, but none to her father.
Rohter's article stated:

Her mother, Jane Wood Reno, cultivated an image as
a coarse-talking, hard-drinking, chain-smoking
eccentric until her death in December at the age of
79. A reporter by trade, Mrs. Reno also hunted and
wrestled alligators, was made an honorary princess
by the Micosukee Indians, kept peacocks and
snakes as pets and instilled in her daughter a rever-
ence for the environment.[2]

No wonder she believes the family institution is dead. She apparently came from a completely bizarre one with an alcoholic and foul-mouthed mother who, though revered nature, lived and fought with animals, I thought.

Then it struck me that the President had also come from a broken home, was an abused child of an alcoholic father—a man, who according to a *People Magazine* report, "married early, often and not always legally."[3]

Hillary Rodham Clinton, however, had a different developmental history. *And perhaps a different perspective then,* I conjectured. Hillary's parents, according to all reports, were model upper middle class citizens. According to Donnie Radcliffe, author of *Hillary Rodham Clinton: A First Lady For Our Time,* Hillary's mother and father, gave Hillary the support, values, and motivation, to promote self-esteem and self-actualization—the fulfillment of Hillary's unique purpose in life. In Hillary's words, "just the best parents can give."[4]

So what is Hillary's purpose in life? According to Radcliffe,

> It was the absence in so many American families of that very kind of stability that had troubled Hillary ever since voluntarily baby-sitting for children of migrant families working on farms outside Park Ridge.[4]

Hillary went on to become the staff attorney for the fledgling Children's Defense Fund after graduate school in 1973. Children's rights became her greatest passion in life.

Could this be a similar response to social injustice which I felt so strongly as a child and believe in today as an adult, I considered. I drew additional parallels to the fact my first experience as a professional educator was with the Massachusetts Migrant Education Program. My life's work I have always felt was similarly child centered. As a post-doctoral research assistant at Harvard my passion was the development of the "self-care motivation model" which my colleagues and I tested in the Gloucester public schools—the purpose of which was to empower children educationally to be all that they can be despite the presence of what I have long felt is an epidemic of parent, teacher and peer abuse.

It was not difficult for me then, to understand how and why Reno and the Clintons might be projecting their abuse, loss, struggles, traumas, and/or major decisions about life and social justice on to the rest of the country.

As a respectful student of B.F. Skinner, with a similar longing for the utopia of *Walden II*, I could appreciate the desire to irradicate social injustice through applied leadership. However, I was deeply troubled by the administration's political agenda aimed at exorcising the 'failed' family institution, and the politics and practices being used to achieve a more ideal society.

Another article I read about Reno added to my concerns. In an interview conducted for USA Today, Jeannie Williams wrote:

> Janet Reno, most popular figure in the Clinton administration, seems still marriage-minded, though single at 54.

> "I always wanted to get married and have lots of children when I was young," the U.S. attorney general says... "I always looked for the right person and what I wanted and I hope I can still find (one)."[5]

The attorney general continued her discourse about child rearing and said,

> " The ages of 0 to 3 are the most formative time... when the child learns the concept of reward and punishment and develops a conscience." Unless this happens, "punishment 18 years from now" won't make a difference."[5]

How frustrated and bitter she must feel, I reasoned. Without a mate or the family she dreamed of having, plus the belief that law enforcement—her chosen career—is essentially futile; the futility in her perspective being due to the lack of intelligent parenting, it's no wonder she would believe and openly proclaim the institution of family has "failed." *Now I understand why she and other "children's rights" advocates would be waging an ineffective war on crime by targeting American families.*

The danger of such beliefs is astounding, I reasoned. *The philosophy to which the First Lady and Reno subscribes encourages counseling rather than punishing outlaws. In blaming the "failed family institution" for criminal violence, they blind themselves to the fact that the principal cause of unlawful acts and repeat offenses is that there are more incentives than disincentives to commit crime.*

The Politics and Policies of the HRS

I soon learned that the second committee Chiles appointed Reno to head was his 37-member commission on government for the people. According to a June 30, 1991 article by Charles Fishman in *Florida Magazine*, Reno was most famous for:

> Scolding the new governor, when everyone was still fawning over his new clothes...

At the first meeting of the commission in January,
Reno wondered publicly why the commission for
the people, appointed by the man who sold himself
as the candidate of the people, had 32 white men on
it, mostly wealthy Chiles fundraisers.

"I don't think you have any consumers," Reno said.
"I don't think you have any people among the working poor. These are $3,000 contributors around this
table, not $100 contributors." The governor's reac-
tion? "He just chuckled," says Reno.[6]

*No wonder he just chuckled, I reflected, what she
said was a joke. Who among the working poor can afford
to be even $100 contributors to wealthy politicians? The
fact that she made that comment shows her political loy-
alties are stronger than her moral values.*

*Also, that she felt empowered to publicly chide Chiles in any
way suggested her ties to those in higher political positions were
already very strong.*

The article continued:

Reno went on to head a Chiles task force seeking
ways to make Florida's paralyzed human services
bureaucracy work again . . .

Her commission recommended a range of ways to
rebuild the underclass and the family. . . give prenatal care to every pregnant woman ("every $1 we
spend on prenatal care," says Reno, "saves us $3
later on"); offer child care to working parents.

She thinks much of the chaos her office sees has its
roots in the decay of the family. "I see what happens when other institutions have failed." Her office voluntarily handles child support enforcement
for HRS...

... She's fully aware that people see the justice system as little better than the welfare system. She has plenty of ideas on how to reshape the system, but her experience hasn't hardened into cynicism. Are drugs the major source of crime in Miami? Then where's the drug treatment? "Treatment," she says, "is a lot cheaper than prison."[6]

I agree with your position on prenatal care Janet, I thought, *but you're out to lunch on the issue of drugs. Drugs are not the major source of crime in Miami or elsewhere, people are—people like you who don't put criminals and drug dealers away to protect people with low self-esteem from succumbing to this form of self-abuse. Given your own assessment that counseling and punishment efforts are futile after age 3, why haven't "children's rights" advocates called for mandatory preventive education programs to train parents to nurture rather than violate self-esteem in their children?*

Then a few other questions for Janet Reno darted through my mind. *If David Acer was alive to stand trial, and was found guilty, would you counsel or execute him? Sure, he may have had his childhood innocence violated, he too was a victim, but how many innocent people end up being the victims of "criminal rights" as well as "children's rights"—the victims of "deadly innocence"— the victims of yours and Hillary's deadly intelligence?*

My internal dialogue continued to express my anger. *I realize that treatment may be a lot cheaper than incarceration, but the death penalty is a lot cheaper than both of these options. Why tax honest and hard working Americans socially with criminal recidivism, and economically with the cost to build and maintain more prisons? But of course, you're making more money with these also, aren't you?*

These questions and others filled my head and directed Jackie's and my dialogue for the next several days. We spent much of that time in our den, reading dozens of Florida newspaper reports published between 1987 and 1992 which Gordon had sent citing the HRS's abysmal record as a social service provider. Jackie frequently joined me, supporting my effort to organize the materials and document the information. As I finished reading an article, I passed them on to Jackie for her to compare the dates with the evolution of the Acer tragedy.

"What's obvious," Jackie concluded, "About the time David Acer was reported as an AIDS case by the HRS and CDC officials, the Florida newspapers were littered with reports about child abuse case oversights by HRS investigators."

"Acer no doubt would have tuned in to the messages," I speculated. "Especially since he was no doubt troubled by his traumatic childhood."

On September 7, 1987, the *Tampa Tribune* exposed two basic problems the HRS had been confronting besides funding. The editor wrote:

Child welfare workers seem the least guilty of all. Given their enormous case load, modest pay and less-than-cheerful working conditions, it's a wonder more children don't die from a double dose of neglect—initial neglect by parents or guardians and later neglect by the state's child protection system.[4]

Because of this the editor posited, many truly abused children were slipping through the cracks in the system and ending up dead.

"This probably aggravated Acer even more." Jackie postulated.

Another most tragic concern was HRS records had shown about 25 percent—or 2,425—of 9,700 invalid child abuse complaints filed in just five Florida counties came from people bearing grudges against one another, and most often from parents fighting a custody battle.

As long as petty people continue filing false complaints, the editor warned,

> HRS workers will remain skeptical about the potential for real abuse in those cases, and children will continue to be at risk of suffering from double neglect—neglect by a parent or guardian and neglect by the system.[4]

Hillary Clinton and the Florida HRS Social/ Political Experiment

On September 10, 1993, I sat in the sunshine on our front deck reading my copy of Donnie Radcliffe's *Hillary Rodham Clinton*, looking for some information about Hillary's connection to Reno or the HRS.

Radcliffe wrote that the First Lady's involvement in Florida's child abuse woes actually began in the summer of 1970 as an intern for Marian Wright Edelman, the attorney credited for developing the Children's Defense Fund. Marian's husband Peter had become a powerful leader in the Democratic Party, a former legislative assistant to Robert Kennedy, and chairman of the League of Women Voters' Youth Committee, to which Hillary had been named upon her graduation from Wellesley. Marian had been a hero to Hillary, because of her long-term support for parent and child education programs. In years to come, both Edelmans would join a loyal circle of Hillary and Bill Clinton supporters active in party politics, civil rights, and legislative reforms.

Hillary's involvement was documented by Radcliffe as follows:

Ten years after the Edward R. Murrow documentary about migrant workers in Florida, *Harvest of Shame.* "I just saw so much, such a great need, and felt that children often didn't have any voice speaking for them," Hillary said.

Edelman had steered her toward Senator Walter Mondale's subcommittee studying migratory labor. Mondale had worked closely with Edelman on the Child and Family Services Act, a major bill to provide compensatory education and day care in the earliest years of life. Mondale remembered "some really tough issues concerning the treatment of migrants—housing, health care, nutrition—and tough hearings" going on involving an orange juice concentrate plant in Florida where housing was especially grim...

For Hillary, working with the Mondale subcommittee interviewing migrants had introduced her to "the conditions in migrant labor camps and to the problems posed by segregated academies that were fighting for tax-exempt status under the Nixon administration, and I came back to law school with a growing commitment toward children, and particularly poor children and disadvantaged ones."[7]

A year later Hillary approached Penn Rhodeen, a New Haven Legal Assistance Association attorney, for an associateship. Rhodeen reported that he and Hillary shared the perspective,

" If where a foster child is placed is working out, don't mess with it. If you ask an old grandma and a world expert what's important here, they say about the same thing. It's the whole middle level that's fighting over turf, saving face and often winding up with everything backward."

... Once you start understanding the problem devel-
opmentally, you realized there was nothing worse
that could happen to that child than to be taken out of
that home."[7]

Hillary according to Rhodeen was very aligned with,

" The fundamental moral dimension of the problem—that you should do these things because they
were right and not simply to save a buck." Even
Walter Mondale, "the guy who was seen as the real
champion of children's issues, to the extent anyone
was," upset her at times when he couched arguments "in utilitarian terms, that it was cheaper this
way or the choice was welfare or jail care."[7]

After reading this section, I passed the book over to
Jackie. "Read this. I think you'll be very interested."

Jackie read the several pages I had highlighted and
then looked up intently. "That's amazing."

"The children's rights agenda represents the philosophical and political platform upon which the principal decisions affecting Florida's contemporary social
welfare and criminal justice system were based." I said
awestruck. "The HRS, founded in 1974, in essence has
been the social experiment of Hillary Clinton along with
other high profile child rights proponents."

"No wonder they kept all the embarrassing details
about the Acer case a secret."

Evaluating the Results of a Social Experiment

About the time Acer was initially diagnosed with
AIDS, the Florida newspapers were reporting on the life/
death struggles of thousands of innocent, abused children and parents. On August 15, 1988, the HRS was be-

rated nationally by the *Wall Street Journal* in a cover story. The following month, the *Tampa Tribune's* Editor published a scathing depiction of the "HRS: The State Agency That's a National Disgrace."

> It would be comforting to charge that the (national) expose was an exaggerated description of minor problems in a poorly managed bureaucracy. Unfortunately, just the opposite is true. The ugly incidents described were all too typical of a social services agency struggling to deal with legislative mandates that all too often exceed its resources and capabilities.

> Frequently, children who are supposed to be under HRS guardianship fall victim to its inadequacies. William E. Gladstone, a juvenile-court judge, put it this way: "Children, neglected, abused and dysfunctional within their families, are further abused and neglected by the same government that should heal and protect them."

> In the eyes of *Wall Street Journal* staff writer Martha Brannigan, HRS is a chamber of horrors where "ill-trained and badly underpaid workers must make life and death decisions based on superficial inquiries... They rescue children from horrible homes only to find there are no foster parents to take them. Worker turnover is so high the agency rushes into disastrous hiring mistakes. This year a former investigator was convicted of having molested two young girls he was dispatched to interview about a complaint that they were being abused."[8]

The administration's essentially denied these allegations and their position was summarized by Coler in a statement made to reporters at the *St. Petersburg Times*. Coler defended,

"Too many people have too much adherence to the goal of keeping the family together."[9]

Six months later, about the time Acer was taking steps to sell his dental practice additional newspaper reports appeared citing the HRS's escalating and deplorable rate of false accusations against parents of allegedly abused children. On February 15, 1989, The *Bradenton Herald* noted that:

> In the last six months, 92 percent of the people accused of physical abuse who challenged HRS's findings were found to be innocent.[10]

The same day, national attention was again focused on the HRS when United Press International reported the agency was responsible for the deaths of many innocent children. The report issued from Fort Lauderdale said that a total of 266 children had died over the past two years including:

> 127 children who died in their homes or in state-licensed centers. Of those, 77 died of abuse or neglect, bizarre accidents or other unnatural causes...
>
> Some of the children had been placed under HRS protection, while others had come under HRS review because they were born with severe medical problems.[11]

Nine months later, on Sunday November 12, 1989, four weeks before Kimberly Bergalis was diagnosed with AIDS the *News/Sun-Sentinel* published an updated analysis of previously secret HRS records. Heralded as the first effort to investigate violence in the state's huge social welfare system, the report confirmed:

> 3,754 client deaths, injuries and other serious incidents in HRS-supervised centers, or involving HRS cli-

ents, between 1983 and 1988. The article cited particular inadequacies in the juvenile justice system, and in the care of
the mentally retarded. In addition, the authors reported:

> The Florida Legislature, meeting in special session
> this week, is expected to consider a plan to spend at
> least $20 million to hire more child-abuse workers
> and train them better.
>
> But critics are not so sure that money will wash
> away the woes at HRS—unless legislators make the
> social services community prove it is spending the
> money it gets wisely.
>
> "They say 'we're dealing with a serious problem,
> we're doing good work, give us some money,'" said
> Boston social welfare expert Frank Caro. "You give
> them the money, and nothing changes."[12]

*Apparently, HRS administrators and Florida officials
felt entitled to keep these data and serious operating
problems confidential.* When questioned about the
policy of withholding the failings of the HRS from the
public, Representative Mary Figg, a Democrat and chairwoman of the state House Governmental Operations
Committee stated:

> "We really felt that the public's right to know wasn't
> worth the price of having the internal documents
> broadcast over the radio or across the front pages of
> newspapers."[13]

After reading this Jackie declared, "That says it all
right there."

"That's the same deadly decision that the authorities
and politicians made that created the entire 'deadly innocence' affair and subsequent 'fear of AIDS epidemic'."

While the Bergalis family was holding their national news conference shortly following the death of David Acer, family rights groups throughout the state were campaigning for the HRS to relinquish their power to local police to investigate allegations of child abuse.

Shortly thereafter, the HRS was again rocked by scandal. In early October, 1990, reporters at the *Tampa Tribune* learned that agency directors had abolished the one office charged with overseeing HRS operations due to the harsh criticism it had issued against the agency's programs.

Bob Williams, the HRS deputy secretary for programs, at the time, defended the move by saying the office had been a casualty of budget cuts.

However, the chairwoman of the Senate HRS Committee, who learned of the agency's action from *Tampa Tribune* reporters, said it must be a mistake.

> "They abolished the office? That seems like a radical idea," said state Senator Eleanor Weinstock, D-Palm Beach. "One of the most serious problems we have in the HRS is that we don't have tools to evaluate."

The article went on to say that:

> Last year the HRS evaluation unit was moved from the Inspector General's Office—the agency's high-profile investigative arm—to Williams' program office. He said it was to make it easier for the agency to implement recommendations.

> Evaluators were surprised when they learned in July that their office would be phased out said Nancy Ross, who supervised the unit and is now an analyst for HRS's Aging and Adult Services program.

"I thought we had been doing fairly good work," Ross said.[14]

In 1989 the evaluation unit had sharply criticized the HRS system of contracting with private mental health centers, the report said. Investigators found the HRS had overstated their welfare savings by not considering $18 million in administrative costs.

Williams stated that his office, which oversees program planning, budgeting and evaluations, would contract with outside firms, colleges and other internal agencies to fulfill the Legislature's mandated evaluation requirements.

The report concluded by noting the HRS had recently contracted to pay an outside company $2.4 million for a five-year look at one of their projects. It was estimated that the elimination of 10 jobs from the internal evaluation unit would save $366,000.[14]

"In other words," Jackie concluded, "They paid $2.4 million to save $366 thousand."

"That adds up doesn't it Jack?"

"Right. It kills two birds with one stone—eliminate the risk of exposure by internal audits, and create an opportunity for corporate kickbacks."

"You bet, politics as usual."

While Reno and Chiles were reviewing the corruption and dysfunction within the HRS, scientists throughout the world were openly attacking the conclusions drawn by the HRS and CDC investigators about the Acer tragedy, and Bergalis was openly condemning HRS investigators for not doing a "damn thing" to admit their mistakes or protect the public from similar catastrophes in the future.

Three months later, during the second week of July, Lisa Demer, the *Tampa Tribune's* chief investigator of the HRS wrote several articles on the agency's "ineptitude and indifference" as 16 more children were found killed under the agency's supervision. According to records obtained a week earlier through a lawsuit against the HRS, filed by the *Tampa Tribune*, these new killings along with dozens of brutalizations had been hushed up. Apparently the HRS cleared itself of responsibility in many of the beatings and murders. The authors stated:

> HRS' failure to see its own shortcomings in deaths like these... underscores the potential weakness of having HRS' local staff do secret audits, critics have said. HRS has done that since the July 1989 abuse death of Lakeland's Bradley McGee.

> Before July 1989, the HRS inspector general's office, based in Tallahassee, issued public reports whenever it reviewed the agency's handling of child abuse cases ending in death.

> But officials ordered the 11 HRS districts to review themselves, a month after a caseworker was convicted of child abuse—based in part on an inspector general's report.[15]

The article went on to report that HRS Secretary Williams, defended the agency by saying,

> "We don't have people in the district whose primary purpose is (investigating the agency.)"

> Williams added that problems in abuse and death cases stem mainly from the low pay, inadequate training and inexperience of workers who must

make life-or-death decisions. Besides addressing those concerns, HRS must offer more counseling and other services to troubled families.[15]

The *Tampa Tribune* reporter's initial review of the 4,774 pages of secret documents maintained by the HRS, provided evidence that:

547 killings, rapes, suicides, attempted suicides, fights, escapes, runaways and abusive acts involving HRS clients [occurred] statewide between July and September 1990, the only quarter completed.

And that's not a complete count. HRS officials acknowledged facilities don't always turn in the "comprehensive client risk prevention" reports begun last year to inform top managers of problems. And some cases tallied locally aren't reflected in the state-wide numbers, a review of the documents shows.[16]

This three month period, we realized coincided with the identification of Acer's first three victims, the publication of Acer's open letter, and the reports filed by HRS chief investigators Howell and Witte regarding the alleged accidents.

On July 23, 1991, during the time when most of America was trying to come to terms with the Acer mystery and the identification of Lisa Shoemaker and John Yecs— victims four and five—the Associated Press reported that a law suit had been filed against the HRS by Karen Gievers, a Miami attorney on behalf of six Dade County children. The siblings had been in foster care for five to ten years. Gievers noted, the "HRS is a lousy substitute for a parent" and charged that the HRS had:

Detained children in foster care too long, denying them chances for a normal life. The suit, which seeks class-action status to represent up to 16,000 foster children in Florida, also calls for the restructuring of the foster-care system.[17]

The article noted that children in the HRS foster care system, according to the department's figures, remain in temporary shelters for an average of two-and-a-half years—a year longer than allowed by federal and state laws. A third of the children remain longer than this, many up to ten years.

"Isn't that ironic," I said recalling a passage out of Radcliffe's book.

"What is?"

"Apparently Hillary Clinton had joined Arkansas attorney and Democratic Congressman Beryl Anthony in representing the foster parents of a child for whom the couple had grown to love and care for over two-and-a-half years. The Clinton-Anthony team successfully argued that it was terrible for a child to be left temporarily in a foster home for two and a half years. Hillary apparently got really fired up feeling the foster parents should have the right to keep the child.[7] Five years earlier, she had also gotten angry when she and Rhodeen had lost a similar case despite having experts testify that taking a child from a foster mother would cause long-term psychological harm to him."

"So what's ironic about that?"

"The fact that the Florida HRS, Hillary Clinton's *Frankenstein*, would be tearing tens of thousands of virtuous families and hundreds of thousands of parents and children apart physically, mentally and emotionally, while hardened criminals receive counseling, then are let loose to inflict more pain and suffering on innocent victims—all in the name of social welfare and criminal justice—that's ironic."

Attacking Ostalkiewicz's Extended Family

Three weeks after Kimberly Bergalis testified before congress, as she lay dying in her bed—the victim of an HRS oversight—*The Orlando Sentinel's Florida Magazine* published a feature article about John Ostalkiewicz's fervent crusade against the "HRS' Child Abuse Witch Hunt."[18] Sandra Manthers, the article's author, interviewed several victims of the HRS bureaucracy. Among them, thirty-one-year-old Janet Cambra, and her husband Kevin—two New Englanders who had followed Ostalkiewicz to Orlando to help run his jewelry business.

Soon after they were settled, their 4-year-old daughter came home from her first day-care experience with a three to four inch bruise on her right thigh. The next day Janet complained to day-care personnel to be more attentive. That night the Cambras were under investigation for child abuse by the HRS who's investigator immediately threatened to take away their little girl. This was Ostalkiewicz's introduction to the Florida HRS.

According to Mathers report:

The HRS investigator who visited the couple's apartment that night spoke English that was sometimes hard to understand.

He gave them no printed information about HRS. He told them nothing of the complex and confusing court process they would soon encounter.

And he seemed unmoved by assurances from the family pastor, a nurse friend and Janet's boss that the Cambras were outstanding parents.

Instead, he demanded that Janet show him the couple's bedroom. He asked what they paid for their 7-year-old bedroom set. he wanted to know how much their rent was.

"Then he takes me outside alone and says, 'I think your husband is a violent man. I don't like the way he's talking,'" Janet remembers. "I couldn't change his mind. He gave me a pamphlet on battered wives."

Kevin Cambra, 33, a slightly built, quiet man, has another theory: "I questioned his authority and he didn't like that. He told me he had the right to take our daughter. I asked what right that was.

"To me, it was crazy. This seemed like something the police would be involved in."

But there were no police, just a man with a business card who suddenly was threatening to take their only child.

"We couldn't believe what was happening to us," says Janet. "We've never been in any trouble. We come from a small Rhode Island community where everybody keeps their nose clean."

Before the Cambras' ordeal was over they would live through six months of psychological torture.

Their nights were often sleepless. Their days became a kaleidoscope of endless questions from doctors, unwanted visits from HRS workers, nerve-wracking appearances in juvenile court and a back-breaking bill for attorney's fees.

"I couldn't even bring myself to buy a Christmas gift for my daughter," says Janet. "We were told they [HRS] could take her at any time."

In the end, beyond their bitterness and vindication, the Cambras were luckier than most who tangle with the largest social service agency in the country.

But then, they had something that most HRS targets don't have. They had John Ostalkiewicz, Janet's 38-year-old boss. And he had the determination and money to fight back.

The lanky, boyish president of CJO Inc., a management company for a chain of jewelry stores in New England and Florida, would follow his office manager and her husband into their toughest battles with HRS.

He would become part of their defense team, spending $20,000 in legal and consulting fees in preparation for the four-hour trial that would determine their daughter's fate.

He would put countless business hours into studying and researching the state's child-protection system, from the initial investigation to the final court disposition.

"I didn't know HRS from the IRS," he says. "I had no intention of getting involved in anything like this."

"But I felt responsible for Janet; I brought her here."

Later, appalled by what he had learned, he would form a non-profit organization to do battle against the bureaucratic Goliath he now calls Florida's Gestapo...

Something isn't right here. That thought kept darting through Ostalkiewicz's mind as he sat in the Cambras' living room and listened the night they tried in vain to convince an HRS investigator they had not abused their daughter.

But the investigator warned the couple that if they
refused to take their daughter to an HRS doctor for a
physical exam the next morning, they would be
arrested and the child would be taken.

All this over a simple bruise on a kid's leg?

Ostalkiewicz's uneasiness returned the following
morning when he accompanied the family to a local
hospital. The atmosphere was subdued, the staff
tight-lipped and condescending, he remembers.

"When we walked into that place, we were condemned," says Janet. "We were just going through
the motions. We were guilty from the get-go. No-
body believed us.

"I had to beg a social worker to be in the room when
my daughter was being examined."

And the same, relentless questions kept coming:
"Can you think of any other way this bruise could
have possibly occurred?"

Ostalkiewicz headed for a hallway pay phone and
began thumbing through attorney listings in the
yellow pages.

That's how quickly it took him to become the most
outspoken activist against HRS.

An unlikely role for a diamond broker . . .

It didn't take attorney Jim Henson long to figure out,
as he sat in his Orange Avenue office and listened
to the obviously distraught businessman on the
other end of the line.

Twenty minutes later, Henson, who was no stranger
to HRS cases, was standing in the hospital hallway
shaking Ostalkiewicz's hand. But he could do little
that day to help his new client.

Henson says the HRS doctor who examined the
Cambras's daughter refused to speak to him or allow
him in the room when the Cambras met with the
doctor.

But he wasn't surprised. He says he's seen it all
before.

"I'll catch hell from the judges, but the juvenile
court process is slanted for HRS," he says. "Children who aren't victims, become victims."

The problem, as he sees it, is that professionals who
deal daily with abuse cases, many of them valid,
eventually lose their objectivity.

"You reach a point where you'd rather be safe than
sorry," he says. "Even judges have heard so many
cases, they are immune to the parents' side."

For a month after their trip to the hospital, the
Cambras lived uneasily in the eye of the storm.
Then, the HRS investigator called and asked them
to sign a "voluntary agreement" to attend parenting
classes.

When they refused, he filed a court petition to make
their child a ward of the state.

"It was full of errors and people were misquoted,"
says Janet. "The investigator said our daughter had
bruises in the pelvic area, which wasn't true."

Nevertheless, the Cambras were arraigned in juvenile court in August 1988 because a judge ruled
there was "probably cause" to suspect child abuse.

Their trial would be delayed until December, but
HRS continued to invade their lives.

An HRS worker visited the home monthly and
asked the Cambras to sign papers promising never
to spank their daughter. Again, they refused.

"We were guilty, even before the trial," says Janet. "And HRS held us guilty even after the judge ruled we had not abused our child."

A few weeks after the Cambras won their court case, HRS sent Kevin a letter, stating he had been "confirmed" as the child's abuser.

The couple requested an administrative hearing to challenge HRS. Two days before the hearing was scheduled, HRS changed the classification to "indicated," a now-defunct category that deleted the name of the abuser, but remained in agency computers for seven years.

Janet and Kevin Cambra, still outraged over their HRS ordeal, say they continue to live in fear it could happen to them again.

Says Janet: "Florida is not a good place to raise children."[18]

Mathers's article went on to report that the state agency investigated 182,291 such reports of child abuse in 1989-90.

In 78,385 of those cases—or 43 percent—HRS determined some kind of abuse occurred and removed 18,000 children from their homes.

An Experimental Disaster

Three weeks before the HRS and CDC investigators published their bogus scientific report on the HIV transmissions, Karen Samples, a staff writer for the Ft. Lauderdale *Sun-Sentinel* published an expose citing HRS supervisors as being above the law.[19] She noted that top administrators did not receive the same disciplinary actions that their employees suffered despite being equally accountable for the failed child abuse investigations and falsified abuse records which were made public in a March report by HRS Inspector General Jay Kassack.

The state's chief welfare official in Broward County defended the administrators saying that in many cases, state inspectors misinterpreted actions taken by three top administrators. Two would not be disciplined, Floyd Johnson explained. The third supervisor, investigations chief Therea Parrish might be disciplined, but he had no plans to remove her.

To some observers, his report confirmed what they already suspected: top-level staff are protected at the HRS.

Kassack's report charged employees with falsifying records to cover up mistakes or work that was not done. Kassack also blamed top administrators for intimidating employees and, in some cases, making false statements to other officials. He recommended discipline for the administrators, but the final decision was up to Johnson.[19]

Two days later in the *Tallahassee Democrat*, the HRS was belittled for being:

A child-abuse industry closed to scrutiny. The HRS budget and bureaucracy has grown rapidly due to an awareness rather than an increase in abuse. Increasing bureaucracy has not decreased abuse but has doubled the abuse registry list of names with too many false accusations. Instilling accountability over bureaucracy could be a major contribution to our state budget solution.[20]

The following month, the *Miami Herald* printed front page headlines that the HRS was on the "brink of disaster." The report described the plight of eleven children who were known to have died while under the supervision of the HRS or after the agency had received warnings that they were being abused.

It wasn't supposed to be this way. "The entire child-welfare system is on the brink of disaster," said Bob Williams, secretary of Florida's Department of Health and Rehabilitative Services."[21]

The article went on to list the agencies symptoms besides the mortality of innocent children under state supervised care.

> Swamped with reports of battered and abandoned children, abuse investigators are falling way behind. Even worse: Investigators in Dade, Broward and southwest Florida have been caught faking and mishandling investigative reports.

> One abuse has been confirmed, HRS doesn't have enough counselors to protect children from further harm. The Lakeland foster-care worker looking after Bradley McGee, who was dunked in a toilet for soiling his pants, had 51 other cases. Today, some South Florida counselors have 71 cases.

> "The system is not equipped to protect anybody," said Elaine Abreu, Dade's child-protection investigator of the month for January, who recently resigned. "You always leave something you have to do undone, because you can't get to it. You lose sleep. You worry about these kids 24 hours a day."[21]

The article went on to report that Governor Chiles would be asking the state legislature for additional funding.

> His "investment budget" would hike taxes to pay for more child-welfare workers, treatment for disturbed foster children and programs to keep families together.

> In March, Chiles vetoed the Legislature's budget, which would have reduced workers, family counseling and other child-welfare programs.[21]

The reporter explained how initially the money that the HRS received added more than 400 new case workers. But as child abuse claims kept rising, the state couldn't afford to keep up with the demand. Following a slurry of budget cuts, the number of case investigators dropped to slightly more than initial levels. This left the remaining case workers overburdened. As a result, many began falsifying documents, fabricating interviews, and lying about physician and police interviews.

The article discussed a recent HRS review and noted:

The review, prompted by concerns that overwhelmed or dishonest investigators might be dismissing cases they shouldn't, found that about a third of the unfounded cases hadn't been properly investigated.[21]

HRS: Successful Business or Social Menace?

According to Ostalkiewicz and others, state kidnapping of children is "big business." Kidnapped children in 1990 earned the HRS $92,000,000 from state and federal funds along with payments from accused parents. While accused parents pay up to $725 per month to the HRS, foster parents are paid as little as $296 per month (1990 statistics).[9]

"Family preservation in comparison receives little if anything." Ostalkiewicz submitted. "Adoption receives a one time fee of $2,000; but foster care receives an inordinate amount of taxpayer dollars. Now you know why foster care numbers have taken a sudden upsurge since the passage of the Gramm-Rudman Act cutting social service monies in other areas. 'Triple Dipping' on kidnapped kids is a lucrative state business!"

The greatest losers in this game of politics, social experimentation and high finance are America's children and future.

"The separation trauma children suffer from being kidnapped from their innocent families and shuffled from foster home to foster home is devastating. The same problem exists for children taken from abusive parents under the present system. Foster care commonly destroys children and creates criminals," the family rights chairman said.

One veteran social worker told me that 69 percent of criminals in California state prisons have foster care backgrounds. In Massachusetts it's 60 percent. An ABC special said that a child in foster care is ten times more likely to be abused than a child in the general population. In addition, children in foster care are twenty times more likely to be murdered." Ostalkiewicz continued, "Florida and California are now spending far more to maintain and expand their penal and corrections industry than they are for the education of their children. Society—people like you an me—end up the big losers as the safety and security we once knew is now gone, and interpersonal violence plagues our nation's youth."

He's absolutely accurate, I realized, recalling my reviews of public health statistics. I knew for example that the only segment of American society whose death rate had increased over the past several decades was school age children and young adults—the 15-24 age group. I knew that the suicide rate for teenagers had tripled since 1959, establishing it as the second leading cause of death among adolescents in the United States—10 percent of teenage boys and nearly 20 percent of girls attempted suicide in recent years. I was aware that automobile acci-

number one cause of adolescent deaths because of the high rate of alcohol abuse in high school and junior high. And I knew that homicide was the fourth leading cause of death in children ages 1-14 and the second for youth ages 15-24.[22]

The picture that began to emerge for Jackie and I however was more frightening than any we had ever realized.

"Is it possible that the Clinton/Reno et. al. social experiment—the integration of social welfare, criminal justice, education, and health care into one government controlled system—is what the Clinton administration means when they talk about shifting the nation's economy from military to domestic economy?" Jackie asked in a rancorous tone.

"Why not?" I contended facetiously. "Rather than fighting wars in foreign lands, why not generate our own unrest—turn our cities and countrysides into war zones, promote domestic terrorism by encouraging violence in youth through 'well intentioned' politically controlled agencies like the HRS. Then we can fight countless futile wars—the war on crime, the war on drugs, the war on illiteracy, the war on child abuse, the war on AIDS, the war on cancer, the war on poverty etc. etc.—each one a financial goldmine besides a nifty way to control the population and engage the ignorant masses."

Donnie Radcliffe wrote in her expose of *Hillary Rodham Clinton*:

> Hillary's passion to make a difference in reshaping
> public policies and attitudes about children's and
> family issues, not the least of which was health
> care, had not lessened in the twenty years since she
> was at Yale. "I think that trying to bring about the

kinds of changes that I think are important is a real gift that I couldn't possibly do anything other than try to fulfill the best way I know how."[7]

As the First Lady flew along side Radcliffe on her way to Washington, "the mother, the wife, the activist, the politician, the moralist" remarked,

"The danger in any kind of a capital city or any governmental activity when you've got power," she said... "is that the sense of mission, contribution and service get mixed up, and pretty soon people start going through motions. The pressures that knock you around all the time can undermine your sense of direction, your integrity as a person and even who you are."[7]

Such is the adversity of American politics—a history of good people and intentions gone awry.

Chapter 17.
Conclusions

The Acer case—the most costly and broadly publicized unsolved mystery in contemporary American medicine—has been assumed to be an accident by the CDC. A better explanation that is supported by the logical and scientific interpretation of the verifiable facts is that Dr. David Johnson Acer intentionally infected at least six of his patients.

This book provides scientific evidence that David Acer was capable physically, mentally, and emotionally of planning and executing his plan to select and then infect at least six mainstream American patients with his HIV tainted blood. As documented herein, there is an essentially identical match between Acer's personal, crime scene, and psychological/social profiles, and those of sexual killers and persons who knowingly infected others with HIV. This book also establishes at least three motives for the murders including: 1) deeply seated and intensely felt anger and aggression towards the CDC and the U.S. Public Health Service for allegedly spreading HIV to the gay community, and not creating a cure for AIDS soon enough to save him from being disgraced in the eyes of his mother and from finally losing his life; 2) extreme hostility and resentment towards American society for believing that AIDS was a gay disease and for being generally homophobic, thus making him and other homosexuals feel insecure, persecuted and angry; and 3) though perhaps less important, the guilt that he had remained a closet homosexual who felt too embarrassed and insecure to participate in gay rights demonstrations and equal rights politics.

In his clearly troubled and obviously demented mind, exposing selected patients to lethal injections would satisfy his desire for revenge and reserve for him a place in AIDS awareness and gay rights history.

The evidence contained herein also indicates that the chief decision-makers within the CDC, the HRS, and the Florida state attorney general's office conspired to keep the Acer case a mystery probably to serve several political motives including protecting top public health and political officials from severe embarrassment.

First Lady Hillary Rodham Clinton and Attorney General Janet Reno were the principal philosophical, legal and administrative architects of the Florida HRS, an organization which defines the state's social welfare, criminal justice, and health care systems. As this agency has been designed to serve as a model for reforming America's health care system, it is possible these two public officials knew of the conspiracy to hide the truth about David Acer from the American people.

Since this conspiracy has cost the health and lives of many thousands of people throughout the United States, a congressionally commissioned independent investigation of these indictments is clearly warranted.

Leaders in the Clinton Administration, the Florida State legislature, the United States Public Health Service at the CDC and HRS, and American society as a whole, should reflect upon the entire "deadly innocence" affair, and the meaning it holds for everyone.

The Fear of AIDS Epidemic

Not since the assassination of President John F. Kennedy have so many Americans been so deeply affected by a scourge of fear and confusion initiated by one man and sustained by partisan politics. Parallels to this case could also be drawn to Watergate as a political scandal. The emotional and financial impact on everyone in the United States who fell victim to Dr. David Acer's intentions and the government's desire to cover them up, however, is unprecedented.

The difference between rational and irrational fear is much like the fine edge of a sword. Brandishing it intelligently serves to protect people from harm. Wielding it unconsciously easily kills or maims.

As a result of the government's unconscious wielding of power and fear, vast numbers of people throughout the United States have now decided that a visit to the dentist, physician, hospital, or blood-bank is a life-threatening rather than life and health-saving event.

Recent studies show that prior to the Acer case approximately 13 percent of all Americans were phobic about going to see a dentist and would avoid going, even when in pain. After the Acer tragedy, published reports show that as many as 2 percent of conscientious medical consumers and 10 percent of confident dental patients began avoiding routine preventive and early interventive care due to their fear of getting AIDS and other infectious diseases from their health care workers.

These statistics imply that *conservatively* about 10 percent of 30,000 people will die of treatable oral cancer this year alone because they were too afraid to see their dentists. Add to this the annual mortality and morbidity increase associated with over 2,000 different types of diseases affecting over 1 million irrationally anxious medical patients, and you can quickly estimate that the "fear of AIDS epidemic" has likely been affecting tens of thousands of Americans annually.

This analysis, of course, does not take into account the toll the "fear of AIDS epidemic" has taken on health professional career satisfaction, stress, burnout and drop out, nor the costs to society in terms of escalated discrimination against HIV carriers and persons with AIDS. With over seven million health care workers in the United States, the numbers who have quit their occupations, or turned away needy AIDS patients due to their irrational fear of AIDS must also be staggering. Such are the costs to society of scientific fraud and political corruption demonstrated in this case.

Lack of Overall Leadership

Likewise, it is the conviction of this behavioral science researcher and public health educator that the CDC's shotgun approach to fear-based AIDS education is similarly damaging to the American people. Research shows that people respond much better to carrot versus stick appeals for health behavior change. For years, behavioral researchers have proven that fear tactics are among the least effective in getting people to change risky behaviors. A recent editorial in the *American Journal of Public Health* reviewed the "trends of sexual behavior and the HIV pandemic." Its author Dr. Anke Ehrhardt, Director of the HIV Center for Clinical and Behavioral Studies noted the greatest changes in sexual behaviors have occurred among gay men, particularly within well-organized gay communities. Dr. Ehrhardt noted:

One reason that safer sex has become the norm in the gay community is that, in the face of many tragic deaths, the community mobilized as a sociopolitical force that determined the content of education and prevention. Using frank and affirmative material that never took an antihomosexual stand, it promoted *pleasurable* sexual behavior that was also responsible and safe.[1]

Ehrhardt went on to criticize the CDC's limited and largely failed attempt to educate the public about AIDS prevention without considering the influence of age, gender, and culture.

Echoing this lament over failed prevention and leadership, *The Nation's Health*, the official newspaper of the American Public Health Association discussed the final report of the National Commission on AIDS. The article noted:

As presidential advisors for the past four years, AIDS Commissioners often tackled controversial issues, criticizing the pace of the government's response in reports that read like road maps on how to slow the disease's reach. But the scores of recommendations were often ignored by past administrators.[1]

June Osborn, chairman of the AIDS Commission said,

"The tragedy is compounded because AIDS is preventable. A strong, consistent voice of leadership could have steered courses of action that might have interrupted the relentless continuation of HIV spread. Instead, previous administrations silently tolerated the epidemic's escalation."[1]

Dr. Charles Konigsberg, the director for the Delaware Department of Health and Social Services and member of the now defunct AIDS Commission warns:

"No disease in history has been conquered without national leadership and a swift public health response."[1]

The Commission's final message to the Clinton administration was that leaders at all levels must speak out about AIDS, and:

Essential to the national plan is a responsive public health system with a sufficient number of trained personnel to carry out the primary public health functions of surveillance, assessment and analysis, and prevention.[1]

It's unfortunate that quality surveillance, assessment and analysis, and prevention by public health authorities were all missing during the Acer investigation from the time he was first identified as an AIDS case to the time of this writing.

The Media's Role

While the American news media might wish to claim its innocence as additional victims in this governmental ruse, as the bearer of the deadly propaganda the CDC wished to disseminate, those in the media are also partly responsible for the tragic effects the Acer case has had on the public and health care system. The media has consistently failed to communicate HIV infection risks in an unemotional, intelligent manner. This failure has largely created the deadly and pervasive "fear of AIDS epidemic" and a society more homophobic than ever.

On Tuesday evening September 7, 1993, the CBS Evening News aired a special "Reality Check." Dan Rather reported that the United States government spends between $2.5 and $3 billion of taxpayer money every year on public relations campaigns. The administration directs

10,858 federal public affairs workers to generate a barrage of press releases which target the media and daily impact the news you and I receive. In essence, Rather reported, "critics say too much taxpayer money is being spent by the government to say nice things about itself." After conducting this investigation and writing up its results, I believe you can't trust anything the government reports to the media.[2]

The results of this investigation also indicate that basically everything any Democratic or Republican administration does of any major consequence is initiated covertly long before the news media presents to the public what the politicians want us to hear. It is therefore not news, it is persuasion—the kind that educates people into ignorance in order to drive a political agenda and/or maintain the status quo of political corruption.

The famous American statesman, the late Adlai Ewing Stevenson once said, "Those who corrupt the public's mind are more evil than those who steal from the public's purse." Unfortunately, both political parties are guilty on both counts.

Homosexual and Homophobic Accountability

On a different but related note in-so-far-as accountability for the Acer tragedy is concerned, the homosexual and homophobic communities should also share responsibility for this tragedy. Many homosexual community members not only tolerated Acer's compulsive and aggressive sexuality, but apparently such behavior was commonly accepted by this population as a social norm. Homophobic society on the other hand is directly incriminated in the Acer case. Acer himself targeted this group for retribution.

The fact is, enduring homophobia and indiscreet homosexuality create one another. The negative beliefs and attitudes maintained by homophobics are reinforced by homosexuals who offensively display their passions. Meanwhile the negative behaviors and attitudes held by homophobics reinforce brazen and gauche homosexual behaviors—a languid attempt at establishing self and social identity. The television news media broadcasts it all, in living color before the masses of impressionable viewers whose behaviors are similarly modeled—not after those bearing a balanced view, but after those who maintain the imbalances, fears, and neurosis which ultimately breeds the psychosis as expressed by David Acer. Can you see how combined innocence and ignorance can be devastating and deadly?

Some Practical Advice

Now that you know that Dr. Acer was a murderer, and that government investigators and officials helped to carry out a cover-up for principally political and economic motives, what can you learn from this experience and do to prevent future pains and losses?

The most obvious lesson is that the "fear of AIDS epidemic" is as deadly as the epidemic associated with HIV, and even now, is being reinforced by many subtle messages emanating from alleged experts and authorities. You should be aware that when you hear stories about: AIDS spreading via mosquito bites and toilet seats, doctors or nurses not caring for AIDS patients, dental and medical professionals advertising their HIV-negativity, and health care workers reacting defensively to earnest patient requests for reassurance—all of these experiences promote fear which leads to additional infectious ignorance, premature death and disease.

Additional irrational fallout from the Acer case includes beliefs that, "All health care workers should be required to undergo AIDS testing, and inform their patients as soon as they become infected with HIV." After the CDC's investigation, people began to assume that mandatory testing and HIV status disclosure for health care workers was the right choice.

In February 1987, *Newsweek* magazine conducted a survey asking readers, "Do you think everyone in the United States should have their blood tested for the AIDS virus?" More than half of the respondents said yes. Unfortunately, mandatory AIDS testing and disclosure are far from "magic pills" for stopping the AIDS epidemic. Such laws won't change people's risky behaviors, they would only reinforce existing irrational fears. Ultimately, mandatory HIV-testing would be much more costly and dangerous to society than maintaining the status quo. Here's several reasons why:

An estimated 40,000 and 80,000 people a year become new HIV carriers. If you test the entire population today, a large portion of new carriers will test negative but are in fact positive because of the incubation period.

There are also many false positives. Experts believe for every thousand low risk persons you test, at least twenty blood samples will test HIV-positive, but half will be falsely positive. How would you like to be the one in one hundred who is told you carry the AIDS virus when you actually do not?

Another concern is that mandatory testing would likely scare off the people in high risk groups who are most likely to test positive and be in need of medical care and psychological counseling. Many of these people would be afraid that knowledge about their infection might be leaked and cause discrimination against them.

Besides the above concerns, at $25-$75 per test, it simply costs too much money to periodically test the millions of health care workers and other people considered to be at high risk of exposure. The costs of yearly testing of health-care workers alone could range around $1.5 billion.[3]

James Berry, Editor of the *American Dental Association News* wrote, the case for mandatory testing "might be less compelling if it could be shown that the only recorded transmission of HIV from a health care worker to patients was the work of a demented mind."[4] This investigation and report, though not necessarily proving Acer did it, circumstantially establishes for most reasonable people, that he intentionally infected his patients, that is, committed murder.

Finally, the greatest unrecognized problem with HIV testing—one which is particularly urgent in light of the Acer case—is the need for high quality pre and post-HIV test counseling. Pre and post-HIV test counseling is essential to reduce all the physical, mental, emotional, social, economic, and legal risks associated with HIV testing. Such counseling can take up to several hours and cost as much as several hundred dollars in addition to the blood testing charge.

As David Acer's case clearly shows, if pre and post HIV test counseling is done haphazardly, it represents a monumental risk for the person going for testing as well as for society as a whole. Pre-test counseling is particularly important to determine beforehand how someone will respond to the news that they are HIV-positive. Physicians and professionals who perform HIV tests must identify ahead of time how emotionally prepared or stable a person is as news of an impending struggle with AIDS often causes people to become angry, depressed, suicidal, use drugs, and occasionally commit socially destructive acts. In Acer's case, thorough counseling may have helped to avert the entire "deadly innocence" affair.

After having written this book about an HIV-positive killer, you might think I would be in favor of mandatory HIV status disclosure laws. I am not and the reason for this is based on the overriding conclusion I reached by investigating the Acer tragedy as well as the cost/benefit analysis I considered regarding this important question.

Dr. David J. Acer was a uniquely deranged individual; such people may be found in every walk of life and in every profession. If, because of this one bizarre case, we were to enact mandatory HIV testing and disclosure laws, many people would be harmed for two reasons:

> 1) Mandatory disclosure laws would reinforce irrational fears about AIDS, as HIV-positive health care workers and people would be singled out as a threat to society which they are not unless they are demented, and 2) many more people are likely to die as a result of mandatory disclosure than the law could possibly save. For example, if medical surgeons were made to disclose to their patients that they were HIV-positive, most patients would no longer go to them. They would lose their practices, be taken out of the workforce, and no longer be able to help save lives and help thousands of people heal over the duration of their careers.

If someone wants to use HIV or any other weapon to kill, history shows they will do so, despite laws which make killing a crime. Mandatory disclosure laws will not make people any safer than they are already given the fact that the risk of getting AIDS from a HIV-positive surgeon is 1 in 40,000 (extremely remote) compared to the risk of dying in a car crash on your way to work which is 1 in 4,167 (very remote).

Does mandatory testing make sense given that the Acer tragedy is the only documented case of a doctor-to-patient transmission of HIV—and in this case the dentist intended this result? Certainly not.

The Difference Between Law and Ethics

The fact that public health officials who work for the CDC knew about Acer without doing anything may be explained legally but not ethically or morally. Legally, confidentiality laws in most states forbid anyone from disclosing or discussing a health-care worker's HIV status without written permission. It's correct to assume that the PBCPHU of the HRS felt that their hands were tied legally when Wolfrom notified them about Acer over two years before he infected Bergalis and the others.

The public health and/or Florida State Dental Board investigators did, however, have an ethical and moral responsibility to follow up his case, which beyond a brief interview and counseling session, they apparently failed to do. This breach of ethical and moral standards only became clear in April of 1991 with the drafting of guidelines for HIV-positive health professionals by the CDC. This guideline, even today, is not required by law in most states, but recommends that health care workers learn their HIV-status through voluntary blood testing. Also, the guidelines make it incumbent on health care professionals, if found seropositive, to voluntarily and periodically consult a local panel of experts, including a medical physician and psychological counselor, before performing invasive procedures.

Today's standard, though not legally binding, the CDC admits, can be used by plaintiffs in malpractice suits. The authorities explain that non-compliant health care professionals would be seen as negligent, and thereby could be successfully sued. This is little consolation to the victims and their families, however.

To the same extent, by these standards, those who informed Acer that he might continue to safely practice may be seen as negligent for knowing Acer's severe and degenerative condition, and not insisting he undergo periodic physical and mental health evaluations to assure the public's health.

What should be done to protect people from HIV-positive health care workers who do pose a potential threat? Enforcing the guidelines established by the CDC is a good start. Current guidelines only emphasize the need for expert panels to counsel HIV-positive health care workers and to periodically evaluate their physical, mental, and emotional health status and their health care needs. Counseling following AIDS or HIV-positive diagnosis should be mandated.

Think about it. Health care workers are now required by the "Bloodborne Pathogens Standard" law to take "universal precautions"—very expensive and administratively challenging infection control practices—to protect people from the remote risks of spreading AIDS and other infectious diseases. Wouldn't it make sense to place equal importance on the care and counseling of *known* HIV-positive health care workers? So long as the CDC's expert panel guidelines are not mandated and HIV-positive health care worker compliance with expert panel participation cannot be assured, the entire "deadly innocence" affair could happen again.

Finally, laws must be made and enforced to assure compliance with thorough pre and post HIV test counseling by physicians and others who conduct HIV testing. Had this been done in Acer's case, the public could have been spared all the unfortunate outcomes.

The Children's Rights Movement

Alexander Solzhenitsyn, one of Communist Russia's most outspoken dissidents once wrote:

> To do evil a human being must first of all believe that what he's doing is good . . .

> Ideology—that is what gives devildoing its long-sought justification and gives the evildoer the necessary steadfastness and determination. That is the social theory which helps to make his acts seem good instead of bad in his own and others' eyes, so that he won't hear reproaches and cures but will receive praise and honors.[5]

Most disturbing about the Clinton administration's view of children's rights, social welfare, criminal justice and public health is the notion that these can be administered by government with all its bureaucracy, waste and corruption. Leaders of the family rights coalition such as Mary Pride counter by saying that under such governing,

> All life becomes politicized... The most powerful man simply declares his personal prejudices to be society's new norms, and that is that. We must all conform or lose... We are even denied the dignity of resisting our oppressors, because they are supposedly tyrannizing us out of love, for our own good, and, in the best interests of [all] . . .[6]

As I see it, the essential philosophical difference between the "children's rights" and "family rights" agendas is that of criminal justice. Should criminals be punished or rehabilitated?

The children's rights initiative believes in rehabilitation. As HRS experience teaches, carried to current extremes, this produces rather than reduces interpersonal violence and crime.

In recent months and years, Florida and Dade County in particular has become America's international embarrassment. At the time of this writing, tourism in Florida, one of the state's leading industries, has been so profoundly affected by violent crimes that international public relations efforts to attract more tourists have ceased. Southern Florida and metropolitan Miami in particular is a combat zone and people throughout the world know it.

Family rights advocates on the other hand believe that criminals should be liberally punished. They submit that from its very beginning, the United States was founded on traditional standards of justice which though not perfect, worked substantially better than what we are witnessing today. To prove their point they simply recommend an unbiased review of historical facts:

Was juvenile delinquency and child abuse more or less prevalent before the children's rights movement was established? Were there more murderers, rapists, and child molesters before criminal rehabilitation programs were developed for these offenders? Were divorce rates pushing 50 percent before the sexual revolution, and children's rights? Was chronic unemployment more or less of a problem before we declared a "war on poverty" and developed an army of bureaucrats to fight it? The answers to all these questions is clearly no.

Juvenile delinquency exploded 11,000 percent since 1950.[7] The rate of incest was one in a million or less in 1940.[6] The incidence of rape, murder and other violent crimes were a fraction of what they are today. Few couples divorced and few children were made to suffer this major trauma.[8] The difference claimed by family rights activists is that today, policies are established by corrupt politicians, special interest groups, and aristocratic fads rather than on basic human values. They argue that social security and general economic progress is impossible in a climate of rampant political corruption and constantly changing laws. They recognize the explosion of violent crimes is the direct result of social programs which provide incentives rather than punishment for criminals, and little justice for their victims.

Pride writes:

Our old standard, of "justice for all" instead of health for all, is simple and time-tested. It requires no elaborate, self-interested bureaucracy. Most of all it is fair . . .

Under our old, fairer laws there was no special category called "child abuse." The same laws applied to those committing crime against children and adults...

Murderers of either children or adults received the death penalty. So did those attempting murder, but failing. This made the question of what to do with a murderous father or mother who has been released on parole or probation irrelevant.

Rapists also received the death penalty. There was no question of getting an incestuous father back together with his tiny victim "for the health of the family."

If a parent knocked out a child's tooth, or blinded an eye, or cut off a finger, or some other atrocity, he did not get free counseling and the chance to sob on some therapist's shoulder. Following the spirit, if not the letter, of the biblical injunction to require "eye for eye and tooth for tooth," he was soundly horsewhipped...

Deliberately neglecting a child physically by starvation or other means was considered attempted murder. Since the penalty for murder was death, hardly any of these cases occurred.

Children who ran away because they were being mistreated (like young Benjamin Franklin, who ran away from his brother) were generally not forced to return. This community feeling had a basis in the Bible's "Fugitive Slave Law," which prevented an Israelite from returning a runaway slave to his abusive foreign master. A small number of children ran away out of sheer rebelliousness, usually only overnight... People who tried to alienate children from their families could be sued.

All this adds up to: punishment for genuine perpetrators, and very little actual perpetration. Parents were presumed innocent until proven guilty, as provided by the United States and Canadian Constitutions. In *no* case did the State assume custody. Orphans went to their next of kin or (failing that) to those willing to help. We had no "search and destroy" squads on the lookout for children to increase bureaucratic caseloads. We also had no network of foster parents who were paid for their services. There was absolutely no financial incentive to set up a Children's Archipelago...

Busybodies were not encouraged. Instead of thinking vile thoughts about each other, under the rule of justice North Americans occupied themselves with their own business. Thus, parents didn't have the stress of trying to prove to every community member every day of their lives that they were worthy of keeping their children.

Those were the days when families stuck together, when fathers were respected, and mothers were all but worshipped. I'm not saying that things were perfect—they never will be in this world. But at least the laws didn't *cause* problems.

You might think this sounds like misty-eyed nostalgia, wistfully (and unrealistically) wanting to return to the dear old days. We constantly hear our self-proclaimed leaders saying, "You can't turn back the clock." By this they mean that we should accept their theories on blind faith, rejecting what we know about the past. But actually, they have already turned the clock back—to barbarism and dictatorship.

As it says in the book of Ecclesiastes, "there is nothing new under the sun." I question whether the values of sexual anarchy and institutionalized living compare favorably with the equally ancient values of family fidelity and home life. The first shot down the Roman Empire in flames; the second civilized this continent.[9]

Then I read Hillary Rodham Clinton's words:

"You have to begin to instill in people some sense of responsibility for themselves and others, and particularly adults for children. And go back to some of the tried and true basic ways that we know work better for them. Children need the right combination of attention and discipline and love. And there are too many who are being pushed into growing up too fast and being left to their own devices too early."[10]

How ironic, I thought, to hear Mary Pride's back-to-basics philosophy echoed.

Health Care Reform?

Finally, the "deadly innocence" affair demonstrates that health care reforms designed to combine free market competition and government regulation as proposed by the Clinton Administration and currently being implemented in Florida under Governor Lawton Chiles will fill political and special interest coffers rather than provide optimal health care for all.

While there clearly is urgent need for health care reforms and cost containment, it is clear that the vast majority of U.S. Government officials and policy makers at the CDC know little about cutting costs and assuring health for all. Nor are they willing to pay more than lip service to the most essential, dependable, and successful form of health care and cost control—primary prevention.

The fact that we have known for decades how and why we should prevent disease without making substantial progress in this direction reflects a combined of lack of moral leadership and pervasive political corruption and collusion between government and the insurance and pharmaceutical industries—the two most powerful political action groups on Capitol Hill.

In 1977, *Doing Better and Feeling Worse: Health in the United States*, a landmark publication, was written by our nation's leading proponents of prevention and edited by Dr. John H. Knowles, the President of the Rockefeller Foundation. The book argued decisively that without a principal focus on "primary preventive health care" (the actions people can take by themselves to stop or prevent the signs or symptoms of disease from developing as opposed to more expensive and risky secondary forms of prevention which involve vaccinations, the early detection of disease through examinations and screening programs, or tertiary prevention which involves the treatment of frank disease in order to prevent illnesses from worsening or causing other illnesses) the American people will continue to feel worse.

Knowles himself wrote:

> Over 99 percent of us are born healthy and made sick as a result of personal misbehavior and environmental conditions. The solution to the problems of ill health in modern American society involves individual responsibility, in the first instance, and social responsibility through public legislative and private voluntary efforts, in the second instance. Alas, the medical profession isn't interested, because the intellectual, emotional, and financial rewards of the present system are too great and because there is no incentive and very little demand to change. But the problems of rising costs; the allocation of scarce national resources among competing claims for improving life; diminishing returns on health from the system of acute, curative, high-cost, hospital-based medicine; and increasing evidence that personal behavior, food, and the nature of the environment around us are the prime determinants of health and disease will present us with critical choices and will inevitably force change.[11]

Unfortunately, as with the recent changes at the HRS, the reforms proposed by the Clinton Administration only places government at the center of a completely dysfunctional system, not to save money and lives, but to make money for politicians through special interest group contributions and increased taxes allegedly needed to cover the unmet needs of citizens.

A similar philosophy and plea for primary prevention came across loud and clear in the distinguished 1979 publication of *Healthy People: The Surgeon General's Report On Health Promotion and Disease Prevention* by the Institute of Medicine, National Academy of Sciences[12]—the basic training manual for every public health officer serving today. Thus, it is not for a lack of knowledge that we suffer our health care woes; the knowledge is simply being ignored.

In 1985, I published "The Self Care Motivation Model: Theory and Practice in Healthy Human Development" in the February issue of the *Journal of School Health*.[13] The paper presented an educational prescription for health care which draws attention to the basic processes underlying all health behaviors. The model acknowledges the physical, mental, emotional, social, environmental, and spiritual aspects of health, and defines a five-step educational protocol for achieving personal empowerment. This "optimal fitness formula" can enable people to become consistently motivated and intrinsically rewarded for developing healthier, happier and more productive lives.

When I introduced the model and the concept of personal responsibility for total self-care at a forum of national health care policy planners at an American Public Health Association conference a few years ago, I naively expected it to be warmly received. Instead, the concept sparked a debate from which the experts concluded that if people were to use the model, and consistently practice primary prevention, then they would likely live longer and as a result, probably suffer more chronic illnesses (associated with old age) which are more costly to treat than acute illnesses which claim lives more quickly. Little attention or value was placed on the benefits of improving people's quality of life, or on the economic, emotional, and social gains associated staying healthy, living longer, and being more productive throughout life. The bottom line really was—if we can't make a buck then it's not worth the effort.

As a health care consumer and political constituent you must understand the complicity and greed which earmark the American political and health care systems. Rather than educating people about their innate potential to remain healthy, some health professionals and most insurers, pharmaceutical companies, and politicians commonly use fear—a standard method for manipulating people's behavior. This is how they maintain power and gain wealth. The majority of fears they promote keep their prey, psychologically and emotionally helpless—dependent on them to provide complex and costly solutions for their continuous course of manufactured problems. The best that they can offer is false hope and periodic relief.

Another mode of manipulation and defense used by policy makers is divisiveness. In other words, they apply labels to people and groups who threaten their status quo and use the old divide and conquer strategy whenever they face opposition to implementing their plans. For example, opponents to Janet Reno's confirmation were labeled and rebuffed as "Christian religious groups and conservative Republicans." By doing so, they effectively turn young against old, black against white, rich against poor, male against female, straight against gay, left against right, one religion against another, patients against physicians, HIV-positive against HIV-negative, etc. etc.

All of these activities are designed to win them elections, make them money, destroy their competitors and confuse the masses. They disempower people regardless of the cost to the public's health and well-being and keep people from having a real sense of themselves—an honest perception of their power to make a difference by expanding self-knowledge, self-esteem, self-love, self-control, and self-care. These are the personal attributes which enable people to make optimal contributions to society.

To create a healthier America, we need leaders, not political puppets, who have the courage to place child and family health education where it belongs—at the top of our country's political and economic agendas. Only by building self-esteem and self-respect at home, at school, and at work can we hope to reap the financial savings and personal and social rewards of optimal self-care and healthy human development. This is our only hope for building healthier families, non-violent, drug-free communities, vital states, a stronger and more independent nation, and a more peaceful world.

Hopefully the decisions we make tomorrow regarding everything from whom we elect, whom we believe, whom we trust, whom we test, to whom we avoid, will be wiser than the decisions we made yesterday, and not based on irrational fear, but on a greater wisdom. As Thomas H. Huxley wrote in his 1868 treatise *Science and Education*, "The only medicine for suffering, crime, and all the woes of mankind is wisdom."

Our greatest challenge in the age of AIDS and health care reform, is similar to that which confronted both Huxley and David Acer, that is, who are we as human beings. Without that knowledge—that "wisdom"—we like Acer are doomed. With it we will be immunized for life against AIDS and all the other woes of humanity.

Epilogue

On September 20, 1993 I received notice from the Deputy Editor of the *JAMA*, Richard M. Glass, that my submission had been rejected. One week later on September 27, 1993 a similar notice was received from *JADA*.

I had spoken with *JADA's* editor several days before the notice arrived and he admitted that it would not be possible to publish the report due to potential liability concerns.

Then he encouraged me to submit the identical paper to a colleague of his who was the editor of a prestigious international dental journal which lacked the political and legal constraints of *JADA*.

"Are you going to do it?" Jackie asked later that evening.

"No, I'll pass. Let's let the American public decide the validity of my work."

About a week later, On October 1, 1993, our long awaited *20/20* edition was aired. Barbara Walters interviewed Ed Parsons who revealed to the nation, in support of our allegations, that Acer had questioned him about whether the AIDS virus could live when mixed with local anesthetics. Parsons innocently told him they could.

In addition, Parsons revealed that shortly before Acer's death, the dentist expressed pleasure that he had gotten all of America's attention. Parsons, disturbed by this, then asked Acer if he had intentionally infected his patients. To his dismay, Acer refused to respond. He only said,

> 'You know Ed,.... hopefully at some point in time you will be able to communicate who I was and help them understand what it's like to live with this disease.' He said, 'well no one is going to believe me any, but I'm not a bad man. I'm not a bad man.'

"I told you he set Parsons up to tell his side of the story."

Her eyes glazed over with exhaustion and pride. "We'll tell the whole story," my wonderful wife promised.

Finally, Parsons explained to Walters how he had tried unsuccessfully to inform the CDC about Acer's troubling comments and behaviors. He said:

"I contacted the CDC. They did not respond. They did not call me back... "

"And *no one* followed it up?" Walters questioned.

"No, not at all."

After the show, Jackie and I considered Parsons's admissions.

"What do you make of Parsons reporting he was never interviewed by the CDC or HRS?" Jackie asked.

"Well, either the GAO investigators lied when they reported the HRS investigators interviewed Parsons, or the HRS and CDC officials lied to the GAO investigators who reported their false claim."

"You mean you trust Parsons?"

"Implicitly."

"Let's go to bed. You've done your job, let a special independent investigator or the media take it from here."

Acknowledgments

The author would like to thank the following people for their support and contributions in the development of this manuscript: Dr. Robert Runnells for his devoted effort in gathering and publishing known facts about Dr. David Acer; the administrative staff of the Federal Bureau of Investigation's Behavioral Science Unit; the Ann Burgess and Robert Ressler investigating groups for their contributions to the field of criminal behavioral science; and Jacqueline Lindenbach for her love, support, time and editorial services; and Gary Kerr for his special care and book design. Finally, I want to thank the people who have supported Tetrahedron, Inc., the non-profit educational corporation I have been privileged to be associated with during the past fifteen years.

References and Notes

Introduction.

1. Grace EG, Cohen LA and Ward MA. Changes in public concern about AIDS following CDC Report. *Journal of Dental Research* 1992; AADR Abstract #35;71:110.

2. Horowitz LG and Pearce TS. A survey of patient and consumer attitudes towards sharing infection control knowledge and costs. In: *AIDS, Fear and Infection Control: a professional development, risk management, and practice building manual.* Rockport, MA: Tetrahedron, Inc., 1993.

3. Krantz L. What Are The Odds: A-to-Z Odds on Everything You Hoped or Feared Could Happen. New York: HarperPerennial, 1992. p. 118.

Chapter 1. The Many Victims of Deadly Innocence

1. The phrase "deadly innocence" means the naivete which makes people highly susceptible to being manipulated, controlled, and violated physically, mentally, emotionally, or spiritually by others who consciously or subconsciously wish to harm them and/or inflict pain, fear, or loss upon their victims. The phrase "deadly innocence affair" used in various parts of this book refers specifically to the complete activities and investigations of Dr. David J. Acer, the Florida HRS and attorney general's office, and the U.S. Government's Centers for Disease Control and Prevention (CDC) regarding the mysterious HIV transmissions.

Chapter 2. The Unofficial Investigation Begins

1. Centers for Disease Control. Possible transmission of human immunodeficiency virus to a patient during an invasive dental procedure. *MMWR.* 1990;39;29:479-380;491-493.

2. Centers for Disease Control. Update: Transmission of HIV infection during invasive dental procedures-Florida. *MMWR.* 1991;40;23:377-380.

3. Horowitz LG and Pearce TS. A survey of patient and consumer attitudes towards sharing infection control knowledge and costs. In: *AIDS, Fear and Infection Control: a professional development, risk management, and practice building manual.* Rockport, MA: Tetrahedron, Inc., 1993.

4. Gruninger SE, Siew C, Chang S, Clayton R, et. al. Human immunodeficiency virus type 1 infection among dentists. *Journal of the American Dental Association* 1992;123:57-64.

5. Kelen G. Assessing risk and preventing HIV exposure in the emergency department setting. *AIDS Patient Care* 1990;4:19-21.

6. Altman LK. Rare syndrome differs from H.I.V., scientists say. *New York Times*, Thursday, February 11, 1993.

7. CBS Evening News with Dan Rather and Connie Chung. New York. September 8, 1993.

8. Goldman BA and Chappelle M. Is HIV=AIDS wrong? *In These Times*. August 5-August 18, 1992. pp. 8-10.

9. Kelly M. Woman who is miami prosecutor joins Clinton list for justice dept. *New York Times*, February 10, 1993, p. A20.

10. Ehrhardt AA. Trends in sexual behavior and the HIV pandemic. *American Journal of Public Health* 1992;82:1459-1461.

11. Kolata G. Targeting urged in attack on AIDS. *New York Times*, Sunday, March 7, 1993, pp. 1;26.

Chapter 3. The Official CDC Investigation

1. Ciesielski C, Marianos D, Ou CY, et al. Transmission of human immunodeficiency virus in a dental practice. *Annals of Internal Medicine* 1992;116:798-805.

2. Invasive dental or surgical procedures are those in which the skin is penetrated and blood is drawn or exposed. This would provide the AIDS virus a direct avenue for blood-to-blood transmission, which is thought to be the principal way in which HIV is passed from one person to another.

3. MMWR. Recommendations for preventing transmission of human immunodeficiency virus and hepatitis B virus to patients during exposure-prone invasive procedures. U.S. Department of Health and Human Services, Centers for Disease Control. Atlanta, GA. 1991;40;RR-8:1-8.

4. Gooch B, Marianos D, Ciesielski C, et al. Lack of evidence for patient-to-patient transmission of HIV in a dental practice. *Journal of the American Dental Association* 1993;124:38-44.

5. Runnells RR. *AIDS in the Dental Office?* The story of Kimberly Bergalis and Dr. Acer. Fruit Heights, UT: IC Publications, Inc. 1993.

6. Street Stories, CBS Television Network, May 21, 1992.

7. Lewis DL. The ADA versus Dr. David Lewis. Unpublished report. June 29, 1993.

8. Lewis DL, Arens M, Appleton SS, Nakashima K, et al. Cross-contamination potential with dental equipment. *Lancet* 1992;340:1252-1254.

9. Gerbert B, Maguire BT, Badner V, Bleecker T, Coates TJ and McPhee SJ. Primary care physicians and AIDS: Attitudinal and structural barriers to care. *Journal of the American Medical Association* 1991;266(20):2837-42.

Chapter 4. Why The CDC Ruled Out Murder

1. 19) Runnells RR. Ob. cit., p. 91.

2. Ciesielski C, Marianos D, Ou CY, et al. Transmission of human immunodeficiency virus in a dental practice. *Annals of Internal Medicine* 1992;116:798-805.

3. DePalma A. No conclusion on ways dentist passed on AIDS. *New York Times* June 26, 1991 p. A14.

4. Drake D. AIDS detectives find only more puzzlement. *Philadelphia Inquirer* June 21, 1991 p. 1A.

5. Centers for Disease Control. Possible transmission of human immunodeficiency virus to a patient during an invasive dental procedure.

MMWR 1990;39;29:489-493.

6. MMWR. Recommendations for preventing transmission of human immunodeficiency virus and hepatitis B virus to patients during exposure-prone invasive procedures. U.S. Department of Health and Human Services, Centers for Disease Control. Atlanta, GA. 1991;40;RR-8:1-8.

7. Martin LS, Hudson CA and Strine PW. Continued need for strategies to prevent needlestick injuries. *Scandinavian Journal of Work and Environmental Health* 1992;18 Suppl 2:94-6

Chapter 5. GAO Investigates The CDC and HRS Investigations

1. United States General Accounting Office. AIDS-CDC's investigation of HIV transmission by a dentist. GAO/PEMD-92-31, Washington, D.C. September 29, 1992.

Chapter 6. More Clues Suggesting Foul Play

1. Davis R. How virus was transmitted remains a puzzle. *USA Today.* May 13, 1993. p. 3A.

2. Kidwell D. Sixth dental patient to get AIDS virus fuels murder theory. Knight-Ridder Tribune Newswire Service, June 7, 1993.

3. Tennessee Dental Association. Former surgeon general sees no cure for

AIDS. *Journal of the Tennessee Dental Association* 1993; 73:39.

4. Berry J. Speculation surrounding Acer cases rises. *ADA News* 1993; 24: 1-8.

5. DePalma A. No conclusion on ways dentist passed on AIDS. *New York Times* June 26, 1991 p. A14.

6. Gooch B, Marianos D, Ciesielski C, et al. Lack of evidence for patient-to-patient transmission of HIV in a dental practice. *Journal of the American Dental Association* 1993;124:38-44.

7. Harrell K. Kim Bergalis' dentist injects another teen beauty with AIDS. Globe. May 25, 1993, p. 1.

Chapter 7. The Runnells Investigation

1. Runnells RR. *AIDS in the Dental Office?* The story of Kimberly Bergalis and Dr. Acer. Fruit Heights, UT: IC Publications, Inc. 1993.

2. Runnells RR. Ob. cit., pp. 83-91.

3. Runnells RR. Ibid., pp. 71-74.

4. Centers For Disease Control. Update: Transmission of HIV infection during an invasive dental procedure-Florida. *MMWR*. 1991;40;2:21-33.

5. "PPO" refers to prepaid provider organization, a third-party insurance provider such as CIGNA, the dental insurance plan to which Dr. Acer belonged. Such organizations contract with large employers to provide health insurance benefits, then refer employees who are covered under their plan to health care workers who subscribe to—that is, pay to be a provider for—the service.

6. Runnells RR. Ob. cit., p. 91.

7. DePalma A. No conclusion on ways dentist passed on AIDS. *New York Times* June 26, 1991 p. A14.

8. Runnells Ob. cit., p. 13.

9. Runnells RR. Ibid., pp. 57-59.

10. Runnells RR. Ibid., p. 294.

11. Runnells RR. Ibid., p. 301.

12. Runnells RR. Ibid., p. 307.

Chapter 8. Will The Real Dr. David Acer Please Identify Himself

1. Runnells RR. Ob. cit., pp. 57-59.

2. Runnells RR. Ibid., p. 75.

3. Runnells RR. Ibid., p. 71.

4. Runnells RR. Ibid., pp. 292-304.

5. Runnells RR. Ibid., pp. 77-79.

6. Runnells RR. Ibid., pp. 60.

7. Runnells RR. Ibid., pp. 61-63.

8. The phrase "safe sex" is a misnomer. In the age of sexually transmitted diseases such as AIDS and hepatitis, no sexual pattern other than abstinence or monogamy with a known HIV and HBV negative person is free from risks. The phrase "safe sex" should be replaced by the words "protected sex" or "safer sex."

9. Runnells RR. Ob. cit., pp. 65-67.

10. Runnells RR. Ibid., pp. 67-70.

11. Ciesielski C, Marianos D, Ou CY, et al. Transmission of human immunodeficiency virus in a dental practice. *Annals of Internal Medicine* 1992;116:798-805.

12. Runnells RR. Ob. cit., pp. 296-297.

13. Runnells RR. Ibid., pp. 293-294.

14. Runnells RR. Ibid., pp. 71-74.

Chapter 9. A Mission of Homicide and Suicide

1. Smith C. Under the influence. *General Dentistry Impact* 1992 20:7-10.

2. The President's Commission on Mental Health. "Report of the Task Panel on the Nature and Scope of the Problem." *Task Panel Reports Submitted to the President's Commission on Mental Health, Volume II, Appendix.* Washington, D.C.: U.S. Government Printing Office, 1978.

3. Perris C. "The Genetics of Affective Disorders." In, *Biological Psychiatry*, pp. 385-415. J. Mendels, ed. New York: Wiley, 1973.

4. Burgess AW, Hartman CR, Ressler RK, Douglas JE, and McCormack A. Sexual homicide: a motivation model. In:*Criminal Investigative Analysis: Sexual Homicide.* National Center For The Analysis of Violent Crime, United States Department of Justice Federal Bureau of Investigation, 1990, pp.39-60.

5. 49) Runnells RR. Ob. cit., pg. 61-63.

6. Belloc N and Breslow L. Relationship of physical health status and health practices. *Preventive Medicine* 1972; 1:409-429.

7. Shaffer D. Suicide: Risk Factors and the public health. *American Journal of Public Health* 1993; 83:171-172.

8. Garrison CZ, McKeown RE, Valois RF, Vincent ML. Aggression, substance use, and suicidal behaviors in high school students. *American Journal of Public Health* 1993;83:179-184.

9. Buckner JC and Mandell W. Risk factors for depressive symptomatology in a drug using population. *American Journal of Public Health* 1990;80:580-585.

10 Schaffer D, Gould MS and Fisher P. Study of completed and attempted suicide in adolescents. File report submitted to National Institute of Mental Health, Rockville, MD. April 1992. Grant R01-MH-38-198.

11. Chiles JA, Miller ML, Cox GB. Depression in an adolescent delinquent population Arch Gen Psychiatry. 1980;37:1179-1184.

12. Kendel DB. Substance use, depressive mood, and suicidal ideation in adolescence and young adulthood. in: Stiffman AR, Feldman RA, eds. *Advances in Adolescent Mental Health: Depression and Suicide.* Vol w. Greenwich, Conn: JAI Press; 1988: 127-128.

13. Levy JC and Deykin EY. Suicidality, depression, and substance abuse in adolescence, *American Journal of Psychiatry* 1989; 462-1467.

14. McAlister AL. "Tobacco, alcohol, and drug abuse: Onset and prevention." In: *Healthy People, The Surgeon General's Report On Health Promotion and Disease Prevention, Background Papers.* U.S. Department of Health, Education, and Welfare, Public Health Service. DHEW(PHS) Pub. No. 79-55071A, 1979.

15. Coates TJ, McKusick L, Kung R, and Stites DP. Stress reduction training changed number of sexual part-

ners but not immune function in men with HIV. *American Journal of Public Health* 1989;79:885-887.

16. McKusick L, Horsman WR, Coates TJ: AIDS and the sexual behavior reported by gay men in San Francisco. *American Journal of Public Health* 1985;75:493-496.

17. Runnells RR. Ob cit., pg. 57.

18. Runnells RR. Ibid., pg. 303-306.

19. Brehm MC and Back KM. Self-esteem and attitudes toward drugs.

J Personality 36:299-314, 1968.

20. Walker RE, Nicolay RS, Kluczny R and Reidel RG. Psychological correlates of smoking. J Clin Psych 25:42-44, 1969.

21. Wetzel RD. Self-concept and suicide intent. Psych Reports 35: 279-282, 1975.

22. DePalma A. No conclusion on ways dentist passed on AIDS. *New York Times* June 26, 1991 pg. A14.

23. Altman LK. And AIDS puzzle: What went wrong in dentist's office. New York Times, July 30, 1991, pg. C3.

Chapter 10. Why Did the CDC and HRS Blunder?

1. United States General Accounting Office. AIDS-CDC's investigation of HIV transmission by a dentist. GAO/PEMD-92-31, Washington, D.C. September 29, 1992.

2. Runnells RR. Ob. cit., pg. 136.

3. Runnells RR. Ibid., pg. 251-270.

4. Ciesielski C, Marianos D, Ou CY, et al. Transmission of human immunodeficiency virus in a dental practice. *Annals of Internal Medicine* 1992;116:798-805.

5. Runnells RR. Ob. cit., pg. 173.

6. Collin J. They deployed the AIDS virus. *Townsend Letter for Doctors.* April, 1988 pg.152.

7. Runnells RR. Ob. cit., pg. 115-119.

8. Runnells RR. Ibid., pg. 69.

9. Runnells RR. Ibid., pg. 83-91.

10. Staff writers. Woman apparently got AIDS during tooth extraction. *Washington Post*, July 27, 1990 p. A4.

11. DePalma A. No conclusion on ways dentist passed on AIDS. *New York Times* June 26, 1991 pg. A14.

12. Drake D. AIDS detectives find only more puzzlement. *Philadelphia Inquirer* June 21, 1991 pg. 1A.

13. Runnells RR. Ob. cit., pg. 94.

14. An "Expert Panel" is a panel of individuals who are considered experts in the physical, mental, emotional, social, economic and legal aspects of AIDS and how the disease might affect persons (such as health care workers) who are at risk of spreading HIV or being discriminated against because of their infection.

15. Altman LK. U.S. drafts guidelines for doctors with AIDS. New York Times, April 5, 1991, p. D18.

16. Jacob JA. Dead suspect means no Acer query. *ADA News* 1993;24;15:1-17.

17. Runnells RR. Ibid., pg. 71.

Chapter 11. Where's The Beef? Finding The Hard Evidence

1. Burgess AW, Hartman CR, Ressler RK, Douglas JE, and McCormack A. Sexual homicide: a motivation model. In:*Criminal Investigative Analysis: Sexual Homicide.* National Center For The Analysis of Violent Crime, United States Department of Justice Federal Bureau of Investigation, 1990, pp.39-60.

Chapter 12. The FBI Sexual Homicide Report

1. Burgess AW, et al., Ob. cit., pp. 39-60.

2. Satten J, Menninger K, Rosen I, and Mayman M. Murder without apparent motive: A study in personality disorganization. *American Journal of Psychiatry* 1960;117:48-53.

3. Ressler RK, et. al. Violent crimes. *FBI Law Enforcement Bulletin* 1985;49:16-20.

4. Burgess et al., Ob cit., p. 41.

5. Burgess et al., Ibid., p. 42.

6. Runnells RR. Ob cit., pp. 57-59.

7. Runnells RR. Ibid., pp. 296-297.

8. Burgess et al., Ob cit., p. 43.

9. Burgess et al., Ibid., p. 44.

10. Runnells RR. Ob cit., pp. 61-63.

11. Burgess et al., Ob cit., p. 46.

12. Burgess et al., Ibid., p. 47.

Chapter 13. Motivating Sexual Homicide

1. Burgess et al., Ob cit., p. 49.

2. Burgess et al., Ibid., p. 51.

3. MacCulloch MJ, Snowden PR, Wood PJW and Mills HE. Sadistic fantasy, sadistic behaviour and offending. *British Journal of Psychiatry* 1983;143:20-29.

4. Pynoos RS and Eth S. Children traumatized by witnessing acts of personal violence: Homicide, rape, or suicidal behavior. In S. Eth & R.S. Pynoos (Eds.), *Post-traumatic stress disorders in children* (pp. 17-44). Washington, DC: American Psychiatric Press, 1985.

5. Burgess et al., Ob. cit., pp. 52-53.

6. Staff reporters. Kim Bergalis' dentist injects another teen beauty with AIDS virus. *The Globe*, May 25, 1993.

7. American Broadcasting Company Television Network, *20/20*. October 1, 1993.

8. Burgess et al., Ob. cit., p. 54.

9. Runnells RR. Ob. cit., p. 71.

10. Runnells RR. Ibid., pp. 260-263.

11. Burgess et al., Ob. cit., p. 55.

12. Burgess et al., Ibid., p. 56.

Chapter 14. Matching Acer's Personal and Crime Scene Profiles

1. Runnells RR. Ob. cit., p. 301.

2. Runnells RR. Ibid., pp. 296-297.

3. Runnells RR. Ibid., p. 13.

4. Runnells RR. Ibid., p. 294.

5. Runnells RR. Ibid., p. 307.

6. Runnells RR. Ibid., pp. 57-59.

7. Runnells RR. Ibid., pg. 60.

8. Runnells RR. Ibid., pg. 53-63.

9. Runnells RR. Ibid., pg. 71-74.

10. Runnells RR. Ibid., pp. 61-63.

11. Runnells RR. Ibid., pg. 268-269.

12. Runnells RR. Ibid., pg. 244.

13. Runnells RR. Ibid., pg. 293-294.

14. Runnells RR. Ibid., pg. 71.

16. Runnells RR. Ibid., pg. 65-67.

17. DePalma A. No conclusion on ways dentist passed on AIDS. *New York Times* June 26, 1991 pg. A14.

18. Runnells RR. Ob. cit., pg. 94.

19. Burgess et al., Ibid., pg. 56.

20. Runnells RR. Ob. cit., pg. 260-263.

21. Runnells RR. Ibid., pp. 77-79.

22. Burgess et al., Ibid., pg. 55.

23. Burgess et al., Ibid., pg. 54.

24. Runnells RR. Ibid., pg. 79.

25. Ressler RK, Burgess AW, Douglas JE, Hartman CR, and D'Agostino RB. Sexual killers and their victims: Identifying patterns though crime scene analysis. In:*Criminal In-*

vestigative Analysis: Sexual Homicide. National Center For The Analysis of Violent Crime, United States Department of Justice Federal Bureau of Investigation, 1990, pp. 61-81.

26. Ressler RK, Burgess AW, Hartman CR, Douglas JE and McCormack A. Murderers who rape and mutilate. Journal of Interpersonal Violence 1986;1:273-387. Reprinted in:*Criminal Investigative Analysis: Sexual Homicide.* National Center For The Analysis of Violent Crime, United States Department of Justice Federal Bureau of Investigation, 1990, pp.82-96.

27. MacCulloch MJ, Snowden PR, Wood PJW and Mills HE. Sadistic fantasy, sadistic behaviour and offending. *British Journal of Psychiatry* 1983;143:20-

28. Cautela JR. Covert reinforcement. *Behavioral Therapy* 1970;1:35-50.

29. Burgess AW, Hartman CR, McCausland MP and Powers P. Response patterns in children and adolescents exploited through sex rings and pornography. *American Journal of Psychiatry* 1984;141:656-662.

30. Poku KA. Knowingly exposing others to HIV: Four case reports and critique. *AIDS Patient Care* 1992;6:5-10.

Chapter 15. The HRS, Reno and Clinton Connection

1. United States General Accounting Office. AIDS-CDC's investigation of HIV transmission by a dentist. GAO/PEMD-92-31, Washington, D.C. September 29, 1992.

2. Kelly M. Woman who is miami prosecutor joins Clinton list for justice dept. *New York Times*, February 10, 1993, p. A20.

3. Berke RL. Clinton picks Miami woman, veteran state prosecutor, to be his attorney general: Third choice, President appears eager to move past turmoil of Baird and Wood. *New York Times*, February 12, 1993, pp. 1;22.

4. Rohter L. Tough 'front-line warrior': Janet Reno. *New York Times*, February 12, 1993, pp. 1;22.

5. Rohter L. Strong hand, sharp eye in justice dept. nominee. *New York Times*, Tuesday, February, 16, 1993, p. A15.

6. Smothers R. Miami ties treatment, not jail, in drug cases. *New York Times*, Friday, February, 19, 1993, p. A10.

7. Rohter L. Debate arises on record of justice dept. nominee. *New York Times*, Tuesday, March 9, 1993, p. A14.

8. Johnston D. Choice for justice is treated gently: First day of senate hearings finds Reno in command. *New York Times*, Wednesday, March 10, 1993, pg. 1;16.

9. Rohter L. Florida blazes trail to a new health-care system. *New York Times*, Sunday April 4, 1993 pp. 1L;26L.

Chapter 16. The Family and Children's Rights Agendas

1. Associated Press. HRS can't do everything for everybody, task group's chief says. *The Orlando Sentinel*, Tuesday, January 8, 1991.

2. Rohter L. Tough 'front-line warrior': Janet Reno. *New York Times*, February 12, 1993, pp. 1;22.

3. Hewitt B, Maier A, Fisher L, Skolnik S, Ellis D, and Haederle M. Blythe spirit: Bill Clinton's dad married early, often and not always legally. *People.* September 13, 1993. pp. 51-54.

4. Editor. Abusing the system. *Tampa Tribune,* September 7, 1987.

5. Williams J. Janet Reno's wait for mister right. *U.S.A. Today.* July 9, 1993.

6. Fishman C. Janet Reno: A big-city prosecutor who talks like a social worker. *Florida Magazine.* June 30, 1991. p. 6.

7. Radcliffe D. *Hillary Rodham Clinton: A First Lady For Our Time.* New York: Warner Books, Inc. 1993.

8. Editor. HRS: The state agency that's a national disgrace. *The Tampa Tribune.* Saturday, September 17, 1988.

9. Ostalkiewicz J. HRS' child abuse witch hunt. *Family Right.* Orlando, FL: Family Rights Committee, Inc., 1992, p.2.

10. Editor. Abusing abuse law: False charges waste time, smear innocent. *The Bradenton Herald,* Wednesday, February 15, 1989.

11. United Press International. 266 deaths reported in HRS files. Wednesday, February 15, 1989.

12. Bergal J and Schulte F. Fatal flaws: HRS clients are paying the price for gaps in care—sometimes with their lives—how the HRS fails Florida. *News/Sun-Sentinel,* Sunday, November 12, 1989, pp 1; 22-23A.

13. Collie T. Broward County baby dies despite 8 abuse investigations. *Tampa Tribune,* June 7, 1990, p. 12.

14. Demer L. HRS shuts down internal audit office. Tampa Tribune, Wednesday, October 10, 1990, p. 1.

15. Demer L. and Long KH. Secrecy obscures mistakes. *Tampa Tribune,* July 14, 1991, pp. 1;13.

16. Demer L. HRS reports show killings, rapes, suicides. *Tampa Tribune,* July 12, 1991, pp. 1;13.

17. Associated Press. HRS breaks rules with long stays. Orlando Sentinel, July 23, 1991, p. 1.

18. Mathers S. Florida's family feud: This man says HRS destroys families—do you believe him? *The Orlando Sentinel,* Florida Magazine, October 20, 1991 pp. 1-17.

19. Samples K. HRS supervisors won't be disciplined. *Sun-Sentinel,* Tuesday, April 21, 1992, pp. B1;B7.

20. Whalen J. HRS should be accountable. *Tallahassee Democrat,* April 23, 1992. p. 4.

21. Rogers P and Viglucci A. HRS 'on brink of disaster'. *The Miami Herald.* Sunday, May 24, 1992 p. 1;18A.

22. Green LW and Kreuter MW. *Health Promotion Planning: An educational and environmental approach.* Second Edition. Mountainview, CA: Mayfield Publishing Company, 1991.

Chapter 17. Conclusions

1. Staff writers. AIDS commission laments lack of progress, leadership. *The Nation's Health,* August, 1993, p. 10.

2. CBS Evening News with Dan Rather and Connie Chung. "Reality Check: The Government's PR Machine.", September 7, 1993.

3. Editorial. Testing health workers is no way to stop AIDS. *USA Today*, Sept 27, 1991, p. 10A.

4. Berry J. Speculation surrounding Acer cases rises. *ADA News* 1993; 24: 1-8.

5. Solzhenitsyn A. *The Gulag Archipelago*, Part One, p. 77.

6. Pride M. *The Child Abuse Industry*. Westchester, IL: Crossways Books, 1986. pp. 129-138.

7. Postman N. *The Disappearance of Childhood*. New York: Delacorte Press, 1982, p. 134.

8. U.S. Bureau of the Census. *Statistical Abstract of the United States*. Washington, DC. U.S. Government Printing Office, 1983, p. 60.

9. Pride, Ob. cit., pp. 129-138.

10. Editor. Abusing the system. *Tampa Tribune*, September 7, 1987.

11. Knowles JH, Fox RC, Callahan D, Thomas L, et al. *Doing Better and Feeling Worse: Health in the United States*. (John H. Knowles, Ed.) New York: W.W. Norton & Company, Inc., 1977.

12. U.S. Department of Health, Education and Welfare. *Healthy People: Surgeon General's Report on Health Promotion and Disease Prevention*. Washington, DC: Public Health Service, DHEW-PHS 81-50171, 1979.

13. Horowitz LG. The self care motivation model: Theory and practice in healthy human development. *J School Health* 1985;55:57-61.

To order additional copies of *Deadly Innocence* as well as other books and tapes on the subject of AIDS, fear and infection control published by Tetrahedron, Inc., please use the order form below.

ORDER FORM

EA.

CODE	BOOK TITLE	QTY	PRICE	TOTAL
0-10-0	Deadly Innocence		$14.95	$
0-06-2	The Post-Exposure Follow-Up Kit		$129.95	$
0-03-8	AIDS, Fear and Infection Control		$19.95	$
0-02-X	Dentistry in the Age of AIDS		$19.95	$
0-07-0	Post-Exposure Follow-up Forms Packet		$12.95	$
0-11-9	Deadly Exposures		$14.95	$

Shipping and Handling:

		SUBTOTAL	$
1st Item	$2.50	SHIPPING & HANDLING	$
Each additional item shipped within the United States add	$0.50		
International orders	$5.00		
Each additional internation item shipped add	$1.00	TOTAL	$
Canadian and international orders (any value)	$5.00 (U.S. Funds only)		

Name_____

Address_____

City_____ State_____ Zip_____

Credit Card #_____ Expires_____

Payment: MasterCard ☐   Visa ☐

Please make your check or money order payable to: Tetrahedron, Inc. Allow 2-4 weeks for delivery.

Mail to: Tetrahedron, Inc., a non-profit educational corporation, 10B Drumlin Road, Rockport, MA 01966

Telephone orders please call toll free: 1-800-336-9266

Other self-care books and tapes written by Dr. Len Horowitz and published by Tetrahedron, Inc., include the "Freedom From" series of titles listed below. Please use the order form below.

ORDER FORM

CODE	BOOK & AUDIO CASSETTE TITLE	QTY	PRICE	TOTAL
8-64-8	Headaches		$19.95	$
8-63-X	TMJ Pain Syndrome		$24.95	$
8-68-0	Teeth Clenching & Night Grinding		$14.95	$
8-62-1	Dental Anxiety		$19.95	$
8-66-4	Tooth Decay & Gum Disease		$12.95	$
8-67-2	Desk Job Stress & Computer Strain		$14.95	$

Shipping and Handling:

SUBTOTAL	$	

1st Item $2.50
Each additional item shipped within the United States add $0.50
International orders $5.00
Each additional internation item shipped add $1.00
Canadian and international orders (any value) $5.00 (U.S. Funds only)

SHIPPING & HANDLING $

TOTAL $

Name_____

Address_____

City_____ State_____ Zip_____

Credit Card #_____ Expires_____

Payment: MasterCard ☐ Visa ☐

Please make your check or money order payable to: Tetrahedron, Inc. Allow 2-4 weeks for delivery.

Mail to: Tetrahedron, Inc., a non-profit educational corporation, 10B Drumlin Road, Rockport, MA 01966

Telephone orders please call toll free: 1-800-336-9266